Contents

Contents

Introduction

Chapter 1 - Understanding Intermittent Fasting Basics	1
Chapter 2 - Setting Up for Success	21
Chapter 3 - Tailored Advice for Post-Menopausal Women	43
Chapter 4 - Overcoming Challenges & Handling Setbacks	63
Chapter 5 - Integrating Intermittent Fasting with Overall Wellness	83
Chapter 6 - Beyond Weight Loss: Health Benefits of Intermittent Fasting	105
Chapter 7 - Real-Life Success Stories	127
Chapter 8 - Sustaining & Advancing Your Intermittent Fasting Lifestyle	148
Conclusion	175
References	179

A Unique Guide to Intermittent Fasting for Women over 50

Lose Weight, Balance Hormones, Improve Mood & Defeat Aging

Introduction

As I neared my 50th birthday, I began to notice my body changing in ways I hadn't anticipated. Despite maintaining a healthy lifestyle, I found myself battling an unexpected opponent: menopausal weight gain. This wasn't just about fitting into older jeans; it was a struggle that affected my energy, my mood, and my self-esteem. It's a challenge that many of you might resonate with, a turning point that led me to explore and ultimately embrace the power of intermittent fasting.

With decades of experience as a naturopath and healthcare professional specialising in allergies, fasting, and weight loss, I've dedicated a significant part of my career to understanding how our bodies react to different diets and fasting regimes. My journey into intermittent fasting wasn't just professional - it was deeply personal. It became the key to managing my weight and reclaiming my health during and after menopause.

Intermittent fasting might sound like just another diet trend, but for many, including myself, it has been a transformational approach to living. It's not merely about when you eat; it's about giving your body the chance to reset and thrive.

For women over 50, this can mean a significant improvement in quality of life, helping to manage weight, enhance mood, and even reverse signs of ageing.

However, I know that many of you may be sceptical. Fasting? At this stage of life? As fasting is completely safe I am offering you not just the science behind why it works, but how you can make it work specifically for you.

This journey through the pages will provide you with a detailed exploration of intermittent fasting, from understanding the basic principles to implementing a plan that aligns with your unique nutritional needs and lifestyle. You'll gain insights into optimising your eating schedules, what to eat, and how to sustainably incorporate fasting into your life without feeling deprived.

It's important to note that this book is crafted with your specific needs in mind. The challenges and opportunities for women over 50 are unique, and they require tailored solutions that consider hormonal changes, lifestyle adjustments, and nutritional needs.

I invite you to keep an open mind and consider this not just a reading exercise, but a stepping stone to enhanced well-being.

With each chapter, you'll find yourself equipped with the necessary tools and knowledge to make informed decisions about your health.

Remember, you are not alone on this journey. Consider me a friend and guide who is here to support you every step of the way. Together, we can embrace a lifestyle that brings vitality, joy, and wellness into our golden years. Let's begin this transformative journey with intermittent fasting and discover the vibrant health that awaits us.

Chapter 1

Understanding Intermittent Fasting Basics

Do you remember the days when skipping breakfast was considered a dietary blunder? It turns out that this age-old advice might not suit everyone, especially as we age. In fact the concept of 'breakfast is the most important meal of the day' comes from an ad by Kellogg's to sell their corn flakes. My own revelation came when my traditional eating habits and regular meals seemed no longer to fend off weight gain during menopause. This experience led me to reconsider and ultimately reshape my view on how and when we eat, guiding me towards intermittent fasting - a practice as old as time but only recently appreciated in the context of modern science and lifestyle.

What is Intermittent Fasting? A Comprehensive Overview

Intermittent fasting (IF) isn't just about skipping meals; it's a structured eating pattern that alternates between periods of eating and fasting. What makes it particularly appealing is its versatility - IF doesn't prescribe specific foods or caloric intakes; instead, it focuses on when you should eat. This flexibility allows you to tailor your fasting regime to fit your lifestyle, making it a sustainable approach rather than a temporary diet.

Historically, fasting is not a new concept. Various cultures and religions have practised fasting for millennia, often for spiritual purification or ethical reasons. In ancient Greece, philosophers like Hippocrates and Plato praised the benefits of fasting. It wasn't until the early 20th century that scientists began to study fasting in the context of its benefits for health, longevity, and disease prevention. Today, intermittent fasting has been revitalised as a health and wellness strategy, gaining popularity for its simplicity and effectiveness, not just among the health-conscious but also among medical professionals.

There are several popular methods of intermittent fasting, each with its own set of rules and benefits:

- **16/8 Method**: This involves fasting for 16 hours a day and eating all your meals within an 8-hour window. It's popular for its ease and effectiveness in improving metabolic health and is often recommended as a starting point for beginners.
- **5:2 Method**: This method involves eating normally for five days of the week while restricting calories to about 500-600 for the other two days. It's praised for its flexibility and has been shown to improve insulin sensitivity and brain health.
- **Eat-Stop-Eat**: This involves a 24-hour fast twice a week. It can be more challenging but is highly effective for weight loss and metabolic health.

Despite its growing popularity, intermittent fasting is surrounded by myths and misconceptions, particularly concerning its safety and effectiveness. One common myth is that intermittent fasting leads to muscle loss. However, studies show that when done correctly, fasting does not only produce muscle gain if you exercise in a fasted state but is used by bodybuilders to gain muscle. Another misconception is that it puts the body into 'starvation mode', slowing down metabolism. On the contrary, short-term fasting actually increases metabolic rate, thanks to a surge in norepinephrine.

These scientific insights help dispel fears and encourage a more informed approach to intermittent fasting.

As we explore the complexities and benefits of intermittent fasting, remember that this journey is about finding what works uniquely for you. The flexibility and adaptability of intermittent fasting make it an appealing choice for many, especially for women over 50 who are dealing with hormonal changes and looking for a sustainable way to improve their health and quality of life.

The Science of Intermittent Fasting & Female Hormones

Understanding how intermittent fasting impacts hormonal health, especially for women over 50, involves delving into the intricate dance of hormones like insulin, ghrelin, and leptin - all of which play pivotal roles in metabolism and appetite regulation. Insulin, a hormone produced by the pancreas, helps cells absorb glucose to use as energy or store as fat. This process is crucial for energy regulation but can become problematic as insulin resistance might develop, particularly during menopause. Intermittent fasting has been shown to improve insulin sensitivity, which helps reduce the risk of type 2 diabetes and supports effective metabolic function. Ghrelin, often called the 'hunger hormone', regulates appetite and plays a role in body weight. Its levels increase during a fast, signalling the brain to induce a state of hunger. Interestingly, regular fasting can lead to decreased ghrelin levels over time, which might help manage appetite more effectively. Leptin, another hormone, signals satiety and helps regulate energy balance. Fasting influences leptin production, potentially enhancing its efficiency in communicating with the brain about energy status and reserves.

For women navigating the post-menopausal phase, these hormonal adjustments through intermittent fasting can be particularly beneficial. The modulation of oestrogen levels, often a concern during menopause due to its significant fluctuations, can also be positively influenced by fasting. Lower and more stable oestrogen levels associated with properly managed fasting protocols can reduce the risk of oestrogen-linked conditions, such as certain types of breast cancer. Moreover, the enhancement of growth hormone production during fasting periods supports not only muscle maintenance and repair but also plays a crucial role in metabolism and weight management, key areas of concern for many women over 50.

Research underscores the value of intermittent fasting for hormonal balance. Studies indicate that intermittent fasting can lead to improved insulin sensitivity and increased growth hormone levels, which are vital for metabolic health, weight management, and cellular repair. For instance, a study published in the 'Journal of Clinical Endocrinology and Metabolism' found that during fasting periods, growth hormone levels increase, which helps maintain muscle tissue and lipid metabolism, ensuring that the body utilises fat stores for energy, preserving muscle mass and function. This is crucial for ageing women who naturally experience muscle degradation and metabolic slowdown.

Begin with shorter fasting windows, perhaps initiating a 12-hour overnight fast and gradually increasing the duration as your body adapts. This approach not only eases the body into the fasting process but also aligns with natural circadian rhythms, supporting hormonal health. It's also beneficial to maintain hydration during fasting periods and ensure that the eating windows include nutrient-dense foods to support overall health and hormone production. These practical steps ensure that as you adapt to intermittent fasting, your body does so with minimal stress, promoting a positive hormonal balance that supports long-term health and well-being.

Navigating through these changes requires patience and attentiveness to your body's signals. The hormonal benefits of intermittent fasting, coupled with a mindful approach to its implementation, can significantly enhance the health and quality of life for women over 50, providing a foundation for a vibrant, active, and healthy later life. As we continue to explore the multifaceted benefits of intermittent fasting, remember that each body responds differently, and the key to successful fasting lies in personalization and gradual adaptation.

Decoding Autophagy: How Your Body Heals Itself

In exploring the vast landscape of health benefits offered by intermittent fasting, one of the most compelling concepts is autophagy. This term, derived from the Greek words for 'self' (auto) and 'eating' (phagy), refers to the body's method of cleaning out damaged cells, in order to regenerate newer, healthier cells. Autophagy acts much like a biological recycling system, allowing our cells to remove and recycle toxic proteins that build up over time, which might otherwise contribute to a variety of diseases. Understanding this process provides significant insights into how intermittent fasting can be particularly beneficial as we age, especially for women over 50 who are navigating through myriad biological changes.

The trigger for autophagy is stress, and while this might sound negative, the type of stress caused by intermittent fasting is actually beneficial. During fasting, when energy intake is low, our cells initiate autophagy to conserve energy and resources. This is not merely about survival; it's about renewal. For ageing cells, which accumulate more damage over time, the initiation of autophagy is crucial. It helps mitigate the effects of ageing by clearing out the old, damaged parts before they can accumulate and cause cellular malfunction - a key factor in many age-related diseases.

For women over 50, the implications of enhanced autophagy are profound. As we age, our cells naturally become less efficient at clearing out debris, which can lead to inflammation and a weakened immune system. Through intermittent fasting and the subsequent activation of autophagy, we can help our bodies more effectively fight off illnesses, decrease inflammation, and potentially slow down aspects of the ageing process. Moreover, the role of autophagy in skin health means it can also help decrease the visible signs of ageing, contributing to a more youthful appearance and healthier, more resilient skin.

Supporting these claims, a plethora of research has illuminated the role of autophagy in disease prevention and longevity. One landmark study published in the 'Journal of Clinical Investigation' showed that increases in autophagy directly correspond with decreased incidence of neurodegenerative diseases in mice models. Another study from the 'Journal of Cell Science' suggests that autophagy can protect against liver disease and obesity. These studies underscore the potential of intermittent fasting, through its activation of autophagy, to provide a protective mechanism against a spectrum of diseases often associated with ageing. In 2016 a Japanese cell biologist Yoshinori Ohsumi won the Nobel Prize for his research into autophagy which comes from the Greek words for 'self eating'. This happens after 15 hours of fasting but some occurs after just 13 hours and the results are similar to stem cell therapy.

While the process of autophagy might seem complex, integrating intermittent fasting into your life in a way that activates this cellular pathway doesn't have to be. Starting with shorter fasting periods can gently coax your body into autophagy without significant stress. It's similar to how you might start a new exercise regimen; you wouldn't run a marathon on your first day. Likewise, easing into fasting helps your body adjust to new metabolic demands without overwhelming it, allowing you to benefit from the cellular cleaning process of autophagy gradually. This approach not only makes the transition smoother but also respects the body's need to adapt at its own pace.

Understanding and utilising the process of autophagy through intermittent fasting offers a promising avenue for enhancing health and vitality, especially pertinent for women over 50 looking to optimise their wellness in later life. The science behind autophagy and its implications for ageing, immune health, and disease prevention provides a powerful incentive to consider intermittent fasting not just as a dietary adjustment, but as an integral part of a holistic approach to healthy ageing. By fostering our body's natural regeneration mechanisms, we empower ourselves to lead a life not just longer, but fuller and healthier in every respect. This knowledge, paired with actionable fasting strategies, can transform the way we approach our health as we age, shifting from a reactive to a proactive stance in managing our well-being.

Metabolic Changes After 50: What Women Should Know

As we age, particularly after reaching the half-century mark, our bodies undergo a series of natural transformations that can significantly impact our metabolic health. For many women, turning 50 is a milestone that often coincides with the onset of menopause and related hormonal changes, which can lead to a slower metabolism and alterations in body composition. Typically, muscle mass decreases and fat takes its place, particularly around the abdomen. This shift not only affects how we look but also how our bodies process foods and regulate weight and energy. Understanding these changes is crucial, not just for adapting our diet but also for embracing practices like intermittent fasting that can effectively counteract these age-related shifts.

Intermittent fasting, with its inherent flexibility and health benefits, offers a practical solution to these metabolic changes. It promotes what is known as metabolic flexibility - the body's ability to switch between burning carbs and fats for energy efficiently. This switching is crucial for maintaining energy balance and managing weight, especially as our bodies become less effective at processing glucose after meals due to a slower metabolism. Moreover, intermittent fasting enhances mitochondrial health, which is vital since mitochondria are the energy powerhouses of our cells. As we age, mitochondrial function tends to decline, a key contributor to decreased energy levels and increased oxidative stress that can lead to chronic diseases. By adopting intermittent fasting, we essentially encourage our bodies to improve the efficiency of our mitochondria, promoting better energy utilisation and healthier ageing.

The strategic approach to weight management through intermittent fasting can be particularly empowering for women over 50. Unlike many diets that focus on rapid weight loss with drastic reductions in calorie intake, intermittent fasting emphasises when to eat rather than what to eat. This focus helps manage weight sustainably without the feelings of deprivation or intense hunger that many diets can induce. It aligns with our bodies' natural rhythms, encouraging eating during periods when our metabolism is more active and fasting at times when it's not. This not only helps in managing weight but also in stabilising blood sugar levels, which is crucial for preventing type 2 diabetes, a common health risk for women post-50.

Consider the story of Marianne, a 55-year-old school teacher who turned to intermittent fasting as a last resort after struggling with her weight post-menopause. Despite trying various diets and exercise programs, she couldn't manage to keep the weight off. It was not only a physical strain but also an emotional one, as she felt increasingly frustrated and helpless. When she started a 16/8 intermittent fasting regimen, her initial scepticism turned to surprise as she began to see sustainable results. Over six months, not only did she lose weight, but she also reported higher energy levels and better control over her eating habits. Marianne's case is not isolated. Many women find that intermittent fasting offers them control over their bodies in a way that no other dietary approach has.

These narratives underscore the transformative potential of intermittent fasting and the deeper metabolic adaptations it can foster. By adjusting our eating patterns to align with our body's natural metabolic rhythms, we can significantly mitigate the metabolic slowdown that often accompanies ageing. This approach is not just about losing weight - it's about redefining our relationship with food and our bodies. As we continue to explore the intricate dance between diet, metabolism, and ageing, it becomes clear that solutions like intermittent fasting do not just address the symptoms of metabolic decline but get to the heart of enhancing metabolic health and vitality, providing a pathway to a healthier, more vibrant life post-50.

The Role of Insulin Sensitivity in Aging

As we navigate the intricate relationship between diet and health, understanding insulin sensitivity becomes crucial, especially as we age. Insulin sensitivity refers to how effectively the body uses insulin to lower blood glucose levels. When our bodies are insulin sensitive, cells throughout the body can use blood glucose more effectively, reducing blood sugar levels. However, as we grow older, particularly after the age of 50, our bodies often become less sensitive to insulin, a condition known as insulin resistance. This change can significantly impact glucose metabolism, leading to higher blood sugar levels and, if not managed properly, increasing the risk of type 2 diabetes, a condition all too familiar to many in their post-menopausal years.

The implications of reduced insulin sensitivity are profound. Elevated glucose levels, if left unchecked, can lead to a myriad of health issues, including cardiovascular disease, kidney damage, and nerve problems. These conditions not only diminish the quality of life but can also shorten life expectancy. The good news, however, is that lifestyle choices, particularly related to diet and exercise, can significantly mitigate these risks. Intermittent fasting, in this context, emerges not just as a dietary choice but as a proactive strategy for enhancing insulin sensitivity.

Intermittent fasting influences insulin sensitivity in several ways. By limiting the window during which food is consumed, intermittent fasting helps regulate the amount of insulin that the body needs to produce, allowing insulin levels to decrease. This reduction is crucial because constant high insulin levels can lead to cells becoming less responsive to its effects. Research supports this, with studies showing that intermittent fasting can lead to improvements in insulin sensitivity and reductions in blood sugar levels. For example, a study published in the American Journal of Clinical Nutrition found that intermittent fasting decreased insulin levels and improved insulin sensitivity in participants after just a few weeks.

Incorporating intermittent fasting into a lifestyle that promotes insulin sensitivity involves more than just managing eating periods; it also includes integrating other health-promoting practices. Regular physical activity, particularly aerobic exercises like walking, cycling, or swimming, can boost insulin sensitivity. Muscle cells require more glucose during activity, so exercise helps pull glucose out of the blood, lowering blood sugar levels and requiring the body to produce less insulin. Combining these exercises with intermittent fasting can amplify the benefits, as exercise during fasting periods can increase fat oxidation, encouraging the body to use fat as fuel, which further improves metabolic health.

Dietary adjustments also play a pivotal role in enhancing insulin sensitivity. During eating windows, focusing on a diet rich in fibres, healthy fats, and proteins can help manage blood sugar spikes. Foods like leafy greens, nuts, seeds, and whole grains not only provide essential nutrients but also help modulate the release of glucose into the blood, preventing sharp increases in blood sugar and insulin levels. Moreover, it's crucial to reduce the intake of refined sugars and processed foods, as these can cause rapid spikes in blood sugar and insulin, exacerbating insulin resistance.

For many women over 50, these changes require a shift not just in how we eat, but in how we view our relationship with food and health. It's about creating a balance that supports our body's changing needs, enabling us to maintain vitality and reduce the risk of disease. As we incorporate intermittent fasting and these lifestyle modifications, we empower ourselves to manage our health proactively, embracing a strategy that supports our well-being through the years. This approach is not just about preventing disease; it's about thriving in our later years, enjoying life to the fullest with the energy and health we need to pursue our passions and stay active in our communities.

Intermittent Fasting: Diet Trend or Lifestyle Revolution?

In recent years, intermittent fasting has surged from a little-known dietary approach to a widely embraced lifestyle choice, capturing the interest of health enthusiasts and researchers alike. But what contributes to its rising popularity, and more importantly, is it just another fleeting health trend? To answer this, we must sift through the layers of excitement and examine the substantial health benefits and the adaptability that intermittent fasting offers, particularly for women over 50.

Intermittent fasting has often been lumped together with rapid weight loss schemes or extreme health fads. However, distinguishing its deeply rooted principles from transient diet trends reveals a sustainable method of managing health and longevity. Unlike diets that impose strict caloric restrictions or elaborate meal plans, intermittent fasting focuses on timing rather than content. This subtle yet powerful shift in approach offers a sustainable way to improve health without the psychological burden of constant dietary limitation. It integrates seamlessly into various lifestyles, accommodating everything from individual metabolic rates to social and work schedules. This adaptability not only makes intermittent fasting realistically sustainable but also enhances its appeal across different cultures and communities, transcending the typical constraints of more rigid diets.

The long-term health benefits of intermittent fasting are perhaps its most compelling argument for considering it a lifestyle revolution rather than a mere trend. Research consistently shows that proper intermittent fasting can lead to improved metabolic functions, reduced inflammation, and lower risk of chronic diseases like type 2 diabetes, heart disease, and certain cancers. For women over 50, these benefits are crucial, particularly as they face increased risks of metabolic and cardiovascular diseases post-menopause. Furthermore, intermittent fasting has been linked to improvements in brain health, including enhanced memory and reduced risk of neurodegenerative diseases. It promotes mental clarity and cognitive function, attributes that are especially valuable as we age. These benefits underscore the potential of intermittent fasting to not just temporarily improve health but to foster long-term wellness and vitality.

Moreover, intermittent fasting's flexibility makes it a culturally inclusive practice. Unlike diets that require specific foods that might not be readily available or culturally appropriate everywhere, fasting relies on when rather than what you eat. This universality allows it to be adapted across different cultural contexts, respecting traditional eating patterns and local cuisines. Whether it's breaking the fast with dates and water in the Middle East during Ramadan or with a light dinner in North America, intermittent fasting can be tailored to fit a plethora of cultural dietary practices, making it a globally accessible health strategy.

In social settings too, intermittent fasting shows its versatility and sustainability. It empowers individuals to make health-promoting decisions without being socially ostracising. Dining out, attending social gatherings, and celebrating festive occasions can all comfortably coexist with an intermittent fasting lifestyle. This ability to adapt to various social situations further enhances its sustainability and contradicts the notion of it being a restrictive, isolating diet trend.

As we explore the layers of intermittent fasting, it becomes increasingly clear that it stands apart from fleeting dietary trends. Its principles anchor in the natural physiology of our bodies, promoting a return to our roots in the rhythmic patterns of fasting and feeding. For us, particularly women navigating the complexities of health post-50, intermittent fasting offers more than transient benefits; it provides a gateway to a revitalised, health-oriented lifestyle. It encourages us to listen to our bodies and find a rhythm that enhances our health without compromising our joy of eating or the social pleasures of dining with friends and family. This balance is not only the secret to its sustainability but also the reason it can rightly be called a lifestyle revolution.

In embracing intermittent fasting, we are not just following a trend. We are adopting a practice supported by centuries of tradition and decades of scientific research - a practice that promises not just better health metrics but a better life. It's a path that respects our body's natural processes and offers a profound way to improve our health, well-being, and longevity. As we continue to integrate intermittent fasting into our lives, we do so with the confidence that this is not merely a temporary shift in how we eat; it is a lasting change towards how we live.

Chapter 2

Setting Up for Success

Embarking on the path of intermittent fasting isn't just about deciding to eat and not eat at certain times - it's about crafting a lifestyle that aligns seamlessly with your personal health goals and daily routines. Imagine you are setting the stage for a play where every element, from the lighting to the props, is positioned perfectly to support the story's success. Similarly, setting up your intermittent fasting plan requires understanding the nuances of your daily life and preparing your body and mind for a new way of interacting with food that enhances your health without disrupting your life's rhythm.

Choosing the Right Fasting Plan for Your Lifestyle

The first step in your intermittent fasting journey is to assess your daily routine critically. Reflect on your typical day: When do you wake up? Are you an early riser who loves breakfast, or do you find your first hunger pangs hitting later in the morning? How about your social obligations and work commitments - do they involve dinners or social gatherings that you would prefer to enjoy without worrying about fasting restrictions? Understanding these patterns will guide you in choosing a fasting schedule that feels natural and sustainable rather than one that feels like a constant battle against your inherent daily rhythms.

Now, let's compare some popular fasting methods to find the best fit for your lifestyle. The 16/8 method, where you fast for 16 hours and eat during an 8-hour window, is widely favoured for its simplicity and effectiveness. It's particularly accommodating if you can delay breakfast or dine early in the evening. Alternatively, the 24-hour fast, known as the Eat-Stop-Eat method, involves fasting from dinner one day to dinner the next day once or twice a week. This method can be powerful for weight loss and metabolic health but requires a bit more mental preparation and resilience. Lastly, the alternate-day fasting method, where you alternate between normal eating days and fasting days, can offer flexibility and significant health benefits but might be challenging to sustain if you have a dynamic social and family life.

Customization is key. You might start with a 16/8 method but find that adjusting the window to 14/10 (fasting for 14 hours and eating for 10) suits your body's responses and daily schedule better. Or perhaps you begin with the Eat-Stop-Eat method but discover that shorter, more frequent fasts maintain your energy levels and fit better with your lifestyle. The goal is to tailor the fasting method so that it enhances your life, not complicates it. Listen to your body and be willing to adapt your approach as you learn what makes you feel best.

Adjusting to intermittent fasting is like acclimating to a new climate - it should be gradual and thoughtful. If you are new to fasting, start with shorter fasting periods and slowly extend them. This gradual adaptation can help mitigate initial discomforts such as hunger pangs and fatigue, making the transition smoother. Just as you wouldn't expect to run a marathon without training, don't expect to jump into a full fasting schedule without giving your body time to adjust to these new eating patterns. Starting slowly not only helps to prevent feelings of overwhelm but also integrates fasting into your lifestyle in a way that feels like a natural progression rather than a drastic change.

Creating Your Intermittent Fasting Schedule

As you embark on this new approach to eating, it's essential to plan ahead to ensure your intermittent fasting integrates smoothly into your week. Think of this as sketching a weekly planner where you pencil in not only your commitments like meetings or family gatherings but also clearly mark your eating and fasting periods. This foresight can be particularly helpful if you have a dynamic week ahead. Planning allows you to foresee and manage potential challenges - such as a late social dinner - that could disrupt your fasting schedule. By anticipating these events, you can adjust your fasting hours in advance, ensuring you maintain the rhythm without stress. For instance, if you know you have brunch on Sunday, you might shift your eating window to earlier in the day and adjust preceding or following days slightly to accommodate this.

Aligning your fasting schedule with your body's natural circadian rhythms can further enhance the benefits of your intermittent fasting plan. Our bodies are designed to sync with the earth's natural cycles - eating during the day when we are most active and fasting through the night as we rest. Optimising your eating schedule to align with daylight hours can improve your metabolism and energy levels, and even help you sleep better.

It's beneficial to finish your last meal a few hours before bedtime to give your body ample time to digest. This can help decrease disruptions to your sleep, as your body isn't working overtime digesting food when it should be resting and repairing. A practical tip is to aim to have dinner around sunset, which not only aligns with circadian rhythms but also can help prevent the temptation of late-night snacking that can disrupt both sleep patterns and insulin levels.

In our modern world, technology offers a plethora of tools that can support your intermittent fasting routine. Many apps and digital tools are designed to track fasting windows and remind you of scheduled meal times, taking much of the guesswork out of the equation. For instance, apps like 'Zero' or 'Fastic' track your fasting hours and provide you with a timer, daily goals, and progress over time. They can be incredibly helpful, especially when you are still getting used to a new eating pattern. These tools also often include educational resources that can deepen your understanding of intermittent fasting and its effects on the body, enriching your experience and commitment to this lifestyle change. Flexibility is a cornerstone of any sustainable health plan, and intermittent fasting is no exception. Life is unpredictable - illness, travel, and unexpected events can disrupt even the best-laid plans.

When these situations arise, it's important to adjust your fasting schedule as needed. If you are feeling under the weather or find yourself out of town and out of your normal routine, it may be necessary to ease up on your fasting regimen. Listen to your body - if you need to shorten your fasting window or skip it altogether to accommodate life's curveballs, do so without guilt. Flexibility ensures that intermittent fasting remains a beneficial and sustainable part of your life, rather than a rigid rule that adds stress.

By planning your week in advance, aligning your eating schedule with natural rhythms, utilising technological tools, and embracing flexibility, you set yourself up for success in your intermittent fasting venture. This proactive approach allows you to navigate potential challenges with ease and integrate fasting into your life as a positive and enriching lifestyle adaptation. As you continue to adjust and fine-tune your schedule, you'll find a rhythm that not only suits your lifestyle but also enhances your overall well-being, making intermittent fasting a seamlessly integrated part of your daily routine.

Essential Nutritional Needs for Women Over 50

Navigating the nutritional landscape during and after menopause can feel like recalibrating your diet to a new normal. As you incorporate intermittent fasting into your routine, understanding and focusing on your macronutrient intake becomes crucial. Proteins, fats, and lower carbohydrates are the pillars of a balanced diet, each playing unique roles in maintaining your health, especially as hormonal changes alter how your body processes and utilises these nutrients. Proteins are vital for muscle maintenance and repair, an important consideration as muscle mass naturally decreases with age. Including adequate high-quality protein sources like lean meats, fish, eggs, legumes, and dairy products in your eating windows not only supports muscle health but also helps in feeling satiated, making fasting periods more manageable. Healthy fats, such as those from avocados, olive oil, nuts, and seeds, are essential for hormone production and can aid in reducing inflammation, a common issue that can exacerbate menopausal problems.

Micronutrients, though required in smaller amounts than macronutrients, are equally essential, particularly for bone health - a critical concern for post-menopausal women. Calcium and vitamin D are well-known allies in maintaining bone density, reducing the risk of osteoporosis. Dairy products, fortified plant milks, leafy green vegetables, and fatty fish are excellent sources of these nutrients. However, the timing of intake can enhance their benefits. For instance, consuming a vitamin D-rich breakfast can help improve calcium absorption throughout the day, which is crucial when your meals are confined to specific windows. Magnesium, another important mineral, aids in the activation of vitamin D and also plays a role in over 300 enzymatic reactions in the body, including those involved in the control of glucose and muscle function. Nuts, seeds, and leafy green vegetables are rich in magnesium and can be strategically included in your meals to support overall metabolic health and well-being.

Hydration is another cornerstone of effective fasting and overall health, often needing more attention as we age. During fasting periods, your body continues to lose water through normal physiological processes such as breathing and perspiration, even in the absence of food intake. Maintaining hydration is therefore critical to support these functions and aid in the detoxification processes during fasting. It can also help manage feelings of hunger and maintain cognitive function. Strategies for maintaining hydration include starting your day with a large glass of water and setting regular reminders to drink throughout your eating window. Herbal teas and infused waters with slices of fruits or herbs can add variety and enhance your water intake without adding significant calories, making them excellent choices for staying hydrated.

Lastly, when planning your meals around your fasting schedule, it's important to consider how each meal can support your fasting goals and overall health. Incorporating a balance of fibre, healthy fats, and proteins in each meal can optimise satiety and energy levels. For example, starting your eating window with a meal rich in fibre and protein, such as a salad with grilled chicken and avocados, can stabilise blood sugar levels and provide sustained energy, making it easier to manage your fasting period. Similarly, ending your eating window with a meal that includes complex carbohydrates, such as a quinoa and vegetable stir-fry, can ensure that your body has the necessary nutrients to support repair and rejuvenation during the fasting phase. They also are beneficial for a good nights sleep.

These dietary adjustments not only complement your fasting schedule but also ensure that your nutritional needs are met, supporting your health and well-being as you adapt to and maintain your intermittent fasting lifestyle.

As you integrate these nutritional strategies into your intermittent fasting routine, you create a supportive eating plan that not only aligns with your lifestyle but also enhances your health, ensuring that your later years are not just about longevity but about thriving. With thoughtful planning and a focus on nutrient-rich foods, you can effectively support your body through the physiological changes of menopause and beyond, making intermittent fasting a valuable part of your healthy lifestyle.

Supplements to Support Fasting & Health

When you embark on intermittent fasting, it's paramount to ensure that your body receives all the nutrients it needs to function optimally, especially since your dietary intake is confined to specific windows of time. This is where supplements can play a vital role, acting as a safety net that guarantees your body doesn't miss out on essential nutrients, even on days when your meals might not cover every nutritional base. Multi-vitamins, omega-3 fatty acids, and probiotics are popular supplements that can enhance your overall health by filling dietary gaps.

Multi-vitamins serve as a broad-spectrum nutritional backup, ensuring that you receive a range of essential vitamins and minerals that support various body functions from immune defence to energy metabolism. Omega-3 fatty acids, found abundantly in fish oil supplements, are crucial for maintaining heart health, reducing inflammation, and supporting brain function, which can be particularly beneficial as cognitive demands remain high in later life. Probiotics, on the other hand, help maintain gut health, which is vital for nutrient absorption, immune function, and even mood regulation. The gut microbiome plays a critical role in overall health, and maintaining its balance can help mitigate some of the gastrointestinal side effects that some people experience when they first start fasting, such as irregular bowel movements.

For women over 50, certain supplements become even more crucial due to the body's evolving needs. Vitamin B12, for instance, is essential for maintaining nerve health and creating red blood cells but is often poorly absorbed as we age. Supplementing with B12 can help prevent a deficiency, which is particularly common in older adults and can lead to significant neurological issues and anaemia. Vitamin D, another critical supplement, supports bone health, immune function, and even mood regulation. Since the body's ability to synthesise vitamin D from sunlight decreases with age, and considering that many of us live in climates with insufficient sunlight for much of the year, supplementation becomes essential. Calcium is equally important for maintaining bone density, which naturally diminishes during post-menopause.

Timing these supplements correctly in relation to your fasting and eating periods can optimise their efficacy. Fat-soluble vitamins, for instance, such as Vitamin D, are best taken with meals that contain fats to enhance absorption. Similarly, taking probiotics during your eating window can improve their survival rates as they pass through the digestive tract, making them more effective. It's also worth considering that taking certain supplements on an empty stomach, like iron, can lead to gastrointestinal discomfort, so timing them during your eating windows is advisable.

Before you start adding supplements to your diet, consulting with a healthcare provider is crucial. This step is not just about safety; it's about crafting a supplement regimen that complements your fasting schedule and addresses your specific health needs without interfering with any existing medications you might be taking. For example, some supplements can interact with medications, such as blood thinners, or could potentially exacerbate certain health conditions, like kidney stones in the case of excess calcium.

Choosing high-quality supplements is just as important as deciding to take them. The supplement industry is vast and not always well-regulated, which means product quality can vary dramatically. To ensure safety and efficacy, opt for brands that have undergone third-party testing by organisations like the US Pharmacopeia (USP), NSF International, or ConsumerLab. These organisations test supplements to verify that they contain what they claim, without harmful levels of contaminants. Additionally, look for supplements that provide nutrients in their most bioavailable forms. For example,

Vitamin D3 (cholecalciferol) is generally more effective at raising and maintaining adequate vitamin D levels in the blood compared to Vitamin D2 (ergocalciferol).

As you consider integrating supplements into your intermittent fasting lifestyle, remember that they are meant to complement, not replace, a nutritious diet. Prioritise getting your nutrients from whole foods during your eating periods, and use supplements thoughtfully to fill the gaps. By doing so, you ensure a well-rounded approach to nutrition that supports robust health, enabling you to make the most out of your intermittent fasting experience and maintain vitality well into your later years.

Preparing Mentally & Emotionally for Fasting

Adopting intermittent fasting is not just about altering your eating schedule - it's a profound shift that affects your whole being, requiring both mental and emotional adjustment. As you set out on this path, cultivating a mindset geared towards success is crucial. It's essential to harbour realistic expectations and equip yourself with a bounty of patience and persistence. Like any significant lifestyle change, intermittent fasting presents its challenges, and your success greatly depends on your mental preparation. Understand that it's normal not to feel fabulous right away and that your body needs time to adjust to this new rhythm of eating and fasting. This adjustment period can sometimes bring about feelings of discomfort or doubt, so it's important to remind yourself why you started. Keep your focus on the long-term benefits you wish to gain - whether it's improved health markers, better energy, or weight management. Recognizing that each small step is part of a larger journey towards health can keep you motivated and committed.

When it comes to managing hunger during fasting periods - the most tangible and immediate challenge - several strategies can help you navigate this new sensation without becoming overwhelmed. First, it's helpful to identify the difference between true hunger and habitual eating triggers. Often, we eat not out of hunger but out of habit, boredom, or emotional need. By paying attention to these cues, you can begin to differentiate between needing to eat and wanting to eat. During times when you do experience genuine hunger, techniques such as distraction can be incredibly effective. Engage in an activity that you enjoy and that requires your full attention - be it gardening, a creative hobby, or even a compelling book or film. This diversion not only helps pass the time but also shifts your focus away from the discomfort of hunger.

Furthermore, incorporating practices such as meditation and mindful breathing into your routine can significantly bolster your capability to manage hunger. Meditation helps in cultivating a state of mindfulness - being present in the moment - which can enhance your awareness of bodily sensations and reduce the urgency of hunger pangs. Mindful breathing, on the other hand, can help in calming the mind and body, reducing the stress that can often accompany and exacerbate feelings of hunger. These methods not only aid in managing fasting-related discomfort but also enhance your overall emotional and psychological resilience, making you better equipped to handle the ups and downs of lifestyle changes.

The role of emotional support in your fasting journey cannot be overstated. Sharing your experiences and challenges with others who are on a similar path can provide not only practical tips but also much-needed encouragement during tough times. Whether it's family, friends, or online communities, having a support network provides a sense of belonging and shared purpose, which can be incredibly motivating. For instance, online forums and social media groups dedicated to intermittent fasting can be valuable resources where you can ask questions, share successes, and learn from others' experiences. These platforms often provide a space for open dialogue and community support which can be particularly empowering during moments of doubt or frustration.

Lastly, one of the more significant psychological hurdles you may encounter is the fear of missing out, especially during social occasions that revolve around meals. It's important to approach these situations with a strategy that allows you to participate without feeling deprived. One effective method is to plan ahead - consider adjusting your fasting schedule to accommodate special events. This flexibility can help you enjoy social gatherings without the stress of breaking your fasting protocol. Additionally, shifting your perspective to focus on the social interaction rather than the food can also diminish feelings of deprivation. By valuing the company and the experience over the meal, you can fulfil your social needs while adhering to your fasting schedule.

Each of these strategies not only helps in managing the immediate challenges of adapting to intermittent fasting but also strengthens your overall mental and emotional fortitude. By preparing yourself with these tools and perspectives, you empower yourself to embrace intermittent fasting not just as a dietary method, but as a sustainable lifestyle change that enhances your overall well-being. As you continue to implement these practices, you'll likely find that your capacity to handle fasting and its challenges becomes more effortless, allowing you to reap the significant health benefits that this powerful lifestyle adjustment has to offer.

Common Misconceptions Debunked

Navigating through the world of intermittent fasting can sometimes feel like wading through a sea of misinformation, particularly when it comes to understanding what fasting means for your body. Let's clear the air on some of the most common myths that might be creating unnecessary concerns or holding you back from exploring this transformative health strategy.

One prevalent misconception is that intermittent fasting equates to starvation. It's important to distinguish between these two very different concepts. Starvation is an involuntary absence of food that is harmful to the body, while intermittent fasting is a voluntary withholding of food for health reasons. Intermittent fasting is a controlled, deliberate method that gives your body a break from digesting food, allowing it to focus on other processes like cellular repair and hormonal regulation. This break can lead to improved metabolic health, increased fat burning, and better regulation of blood glucose levels, among other benefits. Far from harming the body, intermittent fasting is about enhancing bodily functions and promoting longevity.

Another myth that needs busting is the idea that intermittent fasting causes muscle loss. This misunderstanding is likely due to the assumption that without a constant supply of food, the body begins to consume muscle. In reality, the body first adjusts by using stored fat as fuel. Muscle catabolism, or breakdown, happens only when the body's fat reserves are extremely low - a scenario unlikely to occur with intermittent fasting, which includes regular eating intervals. In fact, studies have shown that when combined with resistance training, intermittent fasting can actually help preserve and improve muscle mass, even during weight loss. The key is to ensure adequate protein intake during your eating windows, which supports muscle repair and growth.

The impact of intermittent fasting on metabolism is another area rife with misconceptions. Contrary to the belief that fasting slows down metabolism, research indicates that short-term fasts can actually increase metabolic rates by up to 14%. This boost is due to an increase in norepinephrine, a hormone that helps the body burn fat to be used as energy. Furthermore, intermittent fasting improves hormonal balance, which plays a significant role in metabolic health. By enhancing insulin sensitivity and reducing inflammation, intermittent fasting can help normalise metabolic functions, making it a powerful tool for maintaining a healthy weight and energy levels.

Specific concerns often arise regarding intermittent fasting for women over 50, particularly around its impact on hormonal health. Some fear that fasting could exacerbate hormonal fluctuations and contribute to menopausal symptoms such as hot flashes or mood swings. However, scientific studies have actually shown benefits, including the potential for improved hormone balance and reduced symptoms of menopause. The key is to approach fasting gradually and mindfully, allowing your body to adjust at its own pace, and to consult healthcare providers to tailor the fasting approach to your individual health needs.

By dispelling these myths, you not only gain a clearer understanding of what intermittent fasting entails but also can embrace this practice with confidence, knowing it can be a safe and effective way to enhance your health. As we move forward, remember that intermittent fasting is not about deprivation but about empowering yourself to live a healthier, more vibrant life.

As this chapter concludes, we've tackled some pivotal topics to ensure you're well-prepared to begin your intermittent fasting regimen. From debunking common myths that surround intermittent fasting to understanding the significant role it plays in promoting health, especially for women over 50, we've laid a solid foundation. Up next, we'll explore how to transition into intermittent fasting smoothly, ensuring you're equipped with practical strategies to integrate this practice into your life seamlessly. This will set the stage for a successful and sustainable fasting experience, geared towards enhancing your health and vitality.

Chapter 3

Tailored Advice for Post-Menopausal Women

As the seasons of life change, so too does the body. Menopause marks a significant transformation, bringing with it shifts that can affect everything from your metabolic rate to your emotional well-being. It's a time when many women notice that what worked for them before in terms of diet and health no longer seems effective. This is where intermittent fasting steps into the spotlight - not just as a method for weight management, but as a potential ally in navigating the complex changes of menopause.

Fasting During Menopause: Benefits & Considerations

Menopause is characterised by a decrease in oestrogen and progesterone levels, leading to the cessation of menstrual cycles. This hormonal upheaval can trigger a variety of symptoms ranging from hot flashes to mood swings, and often a noticeable change in how your body stores fat, particularly around the abdomen. These changes aren't just influenced by hormones; they're also intertwined with shifts in insulin sensitivity, metabolism, and energy levels. It's a period that requires not just medical attention but a reassessment of lifestyle habits, especially nutrition.

Intermittent fasting emerges as a compelling approach during this phase of life, primarily because of its influence on insulin sensitivity and body composition. As oestrogen levels decline, your body's response to insulin can change, leading to increased insulin resistance. This shift makes weight loss more challenging and increases the risk of type 2 diabetes. Intermittent fasting can counteract these effects by improving how your body responds to insulin. During fasting periods, insulin levels drop significantly, which can help to reverse insulin resistance. Over time, this can lead to improved blood sugar control, reduced inflammation, and even weight loss -

outcomes that are often harder to achieve during and after menopause through diet alone.

Moreover, intermittent fasting activates cellular mechanisms that go beyond simple weight management. One of these mechanisms is autophagy, a process that helps clear out damaged cells and regenerate new ones. This cellular cleanup is particularly beneficial as you age, helping to counteract the accumulation of cellular damage linked to ageing and menopause. The increased fat burning and energy efficiency provided by intermittent fasting can also help manage and mitigate common menopausal symptoms, providing a more stable energy base throughout the day.

Choosing the right fasting window is crucial, particularly during menopause. Your body's tolerance for long fasting periods might change, and what once felt manageable might now feel overwhelming. Start with shorter fasting windows, perhaps the 16/8 method, and adjust according to how your body responds. Some women find that fasting through the morning and breaking their fast around midday suits their hormonal fluctuations better, particularly if they experience morning sluggishness. It's also important to consider your lifestyle and energy demands - choosing a fasting schedule that disrupts your sleep or daily activities is unlikely to be sustainable.

Listening to your body is more than a cliché during menopause - it's essential. Your body's signals might change: what hunger and fullness felt like before might not be the same now. You might also find your energy levels fluctuating more than usual. Adjusting your fasting and eating windows to accommodate these changes is not just about maintaining comfort but about enhancing the efficacy of your fasting regimen. If you find that certain fasting schedules exacerbate menopausal symptoms like fatigue or irritability, it's a sign to reassess and modify your approach. Remember, the goal of intermittent fasting during menopause isn't just to adhere to a schedule, but to find a rhythm that harmonises with your body's needs during this transformative period.

In this chapter, we delve deeper into how intermittent fasting can be specifically tailored to the needs and challenges faced by post-menopausal women. By understanding the physiological changes unique to this stage of life and adjusting your fasting regimen to accommodate these changes, you can enhance your health, manage symptoms, and improve your overall quality of life during menopause. As we explore further, remember that each woman's experience of menopause is unique, and so too should be her approach to fasting.

Managing Hot Flashes & Hormonal Fluctuations

Hot flashes are one of the more conspicuous and often frustrating symptoms associated with menopause, characterised by sudden warmth, flushing, and sweating that many women experience. This phenomenon is largely due to the hormonal fluctuations that occur during menopause, particularly the decrease in oestrogen levels. Interestingly, intermittent fasting may influence these hormonal activities, offering potential relief from hot flashes. The mechanism behind this involves the regulatory effects of fasting on insulin and blood sugar levels, which can indirectly influence hormone regulation and thus, potentially mitigate the frequency and intensity of hot flashes. While the direct correlation between intermittent fasting and reduced hot flashes is an area ripe for further research, the anecdotal evidence from many women who have integrated fasting into their lifestyle is compelling and worthy of consideration.

During the eating windows within your intermittent fasting schedule, certain dietary adjustments can also play a crucial role in stabilising hormone levels and reducing the occurrence of hot flashes. Foods rich in phytoestrogens, such as soy products, flaxseeds, and certain nuts and seeds, can have a mild estrogenic effect on the body, which may help balance hormone levels and alleviate some menopausal symptoms. Incorporating foods high in omega-3 fatty acids like salmon, walnuts, and flaxseed can also be beneficial, as these nutrients help combat inflammation, which can exacerbate hot flashes. Furthermore, maintaining a diet low in spicy foods, caffeine, and alcohol can help manage hot flashes, as these substances are known triggers that can intensify their frequency and severity.

In addition to dietary strategies, integrating stress management techniques such as yoga and meditation into your routine can have a profound effect on hormonal balance and hot flash management. Stress is known to exacerbate menopausal symptoms, including hot flashes, due to its impact on cortisol and adrenaline levels, which can further unbalance hormones. Practices like yoga not only help reduce stress but also improve overall well-being by enhancing flexibility, strength, and balance. Meditation, particularly mindfulness meditation, can help you manage the emotional responses to the discomforts associated with menopause, including anxiety and irritability, which in turn can help alleviate the physiological symptoms such as hot flashes.

Regular monitoring of your symptoms is crucial to effectively manage and adjust your intermittent fasting and dietary strategies to best suit your needs during menopause. Keeping a journal where you track your hot flashes, noting their frequency, intensity, and any associated activities or foods, can provide valuable insights into what might be triggering them or exacerbating their severity. This record can help you tailor your fasting and dietary approaches more accurately, allowing for a more personalised strategy that addresses your specific symptoms. If you notice an increase in discomfort or that your hot flashes worsen, it may be necessary to reevaluate your fasting schedule, perhaps adjusting the duration of fasts or the timing of your eating windows to better align with your body's needs during this sensitive time.

Adopting these strategies requires patience and persistence, but by doing so, you can create a supportive environment that not only eases the physical symptoms of menopause but also enhances your overall quality of life during this transformative phase.

Nutrition Focus: Phytoestrogens & Bone Health

Navigating through the nutritional needs of your body during menopause can feel like a delicate balancing act, especially when it comes to managing symptoms and ensuring long-term health. One of the pivotal elements in this equation is phytoestrogens, naturally occurring compounds in plants that can mimic the effects of oestrogen in the body. During menopause, as your body's natural production of oestrogen decreases, these plant-based substitutes can play a beneficial role in smoothing out the hormonal fluctuations that contribute to menopausal symptoms, such as hot flashes and mood swings. Phytoestrogens bind to the same receptors as oestrogen, potentially helping to moderate the body's response to lower oestrogen levels.

The most well-known sources of phytoestrogens include flax seeds, soy products like tofu and tempeh, and various berries. Flax seeds, for instance, are not only high in phytoestrogens but are also an excellent source of fibre and omega-3 fatty acids, which support heart health and reduce inflammation. Incorporating these into your diet can be as simple as adding a tablespoon of ground flaxseed to your morning smoothie or oatmeal. Soy products, which contain isoflavones, a type of phytoestrogen, can be included in meals as tofu stir-fries or snacks like edamame. Berries, aside from their phytoestrogen content, offer high levels of antioxidants, which are crucial for cellular health and inflammation control. Regularly including these foods in your eating windows not only provides your body with phytoestrogens but also enhances your overall nutrient intake, supporting broader health and well-being.

Equally critical during menopause is the maintenance of bone density. The decline in oestrogen levels during menopause can accelerate bone loss, increasing the risk of osteoporosis and fractures. Calcium and vitamin D are the cornerstones of good bone health. Calcium supports the structure and density of bones, while vitamin D enhances calcium absorption and bone growth. However, getting adequate amounts of these nutrients can be challenging, eggs and free range meat can supply most of your needs. Dairy products are well-known calcium-rich foods, but if you're dairy-intolerant or vegan, you can turn to fortified plant milks and juices, which can be just as effective. Leafy green vegetables like kale and spinach are also excellent sources of calcium.

For vitamin D, while exposure to sunlight is the most natural way to boost your levels, the reality for many, especially during the winter months, is that sunlight isn't enough. Foods like fatty fish, egg yolks, and fortified foods play a crucial role, and supplements might be necessary to achieve adequate levels. It is important to consult with a healthcare provider to determine the right dosage, as vitamin D needs can vary based on individual factors including age, geographic location, skin colour, and current vitamin D levels, which can be determined through a blood test.

When it comes to meal planning, integrating these nutrients effectively requires thoughtful consideration of your eating windows. For instance, starting your day with a breakfast that includes a spinach and cheese omelette can provide a hearty dose of calcium, while a lunch that features grilled salmon salad can cover both your vitamin D and omega-3 fatty acids requirements. Snacking on almonds or roasted soybeans can also boost your calcium intake throughout your eating period. To enhance the absorption of these nutrients, it's beneficial to include sources of vitamin C like citrus fruits or bell peppers, which can help increase the bioavailability of plant-based iron and calcium, making these nutrients more accessible for your body to use.

In crafting your meals, consider not only the composition but also the timing. Consuming a balanced dinner that finishes with a small bowl of mixed berries can provide a final boost of phytoestrogens and antioxidants before your fasting period begins. This not only maximises nutrient intake but also ensures that you go into your fasting period nutritionally satisfied, which can help manage hunger and sustain energy levels until your next eating window. Remember, the goal of integrating these nutritional strategies is not just to manage menopause symptoms but to enhance overall health, ensuring that you can enjoy this new phase of life with vitality and strength.

Weight Management After Menopause

Navigating weight management after menopause can often feel like battling an uphill struggle. As oestrogen levels drop, many women find that their metabolism slows down, which can lead to weight gain, particularly around the abdomen. This change is not just a cosmetic concern; it has significant implications for health, including increased risks for cardiovascular disease and type 2 diabetes. Understanding these changes and adapting your lifestyle accordingly is crucial for maintaining your health and well-being during this transformative phase of life.

Intermittent fasting emerges as a particularly effective strategy for managing weight during menopause. The process of fasting works to improve metabolic health by enhancing the body's ability to utilise fat for energy, rather than storing it. This shift is achieved through several mechanisms, including improvements in insulin sensitivity. When your body becomes more sensitive to insulin, it reduces the likelihood of excess glucose being stored as fat, helping to counteract the weight gain often associated with hormonal changes in menopause. Moreover, intermittent fasting can increase levels of human growth hormone (HGH), which plays a key role in health, fitness, and slowing the ageing process. HGH not only helps in fat loss but also in preserving lean muscle mass, which can otherwise decline with age.

Incorporating physical activity into your routine is another vital component of weight management after menopause. While intermittent fasting sets the stage for fat loss, physical activity, especially strength training, complements this by enhancing muscle mass and overall metabolic rate. Muscle tissue burns more calories than fat tissue, even at rest, so maintaining or increasing muscle mass is crucial for weight management. Strength training, such as lifting weights, using resistance bands, or performing body-weight exercises, can be particularly effective.

Not only does it help in maintaining muscle mass, but it also improves bone density, which is crucial for preventing osteoporosis, a common concern for post-menopausal women. Integrating regular physical activity that you enjoy and can maintain long-term is key. Whether it's yoga, swimming, or a daily walk, the best exercise is the one you can keep doing consistently.

Adopting behavioural strategies to manage your lifestyle changes effectively is equally important. Setting realistic weight management goals is a critical step. Often, post-menopausal weight loss may not be as rapid or as much as it might have been earlier in life, and that's perfectly normal. Adjusting your expectations to align with realistic, health-focused goals rather than just cosmetic changes can help maintain motivation and prevent frustration. Keeping a food and activity journal is an excellent method for staying on track with these goals. This practice not only helps in monitoring your daily intake and physical activity but also offers insights into patterns such as emotional eating or times when you are more likely to skip exercise. Over time, this data can help you make informed adjustments that better suit your lifestyle and health needs.

By understanding the unique challenges of weight management during menopause and strategically incorporating intermittent fasting, physical activity, and behavioural strategies into your life, you can improve not only your body composition but also your overall health and vitality. This holistic approach ensures that you are not only losing weight but also building a healthier, more active, and satisfying life in your post-menopausal years.

Fasting & Sleep Patterns

The intricate dance between our dietary habits and sleep quality often goes unnoticed until we make a significant change, such as adopting intermittent fasting. For women navigating the post-menopausal phase, understanding how fasting influences sleep is crucial, given that hormonal fluctuations during this time can already disrupt sleep patterns. During fasting, changes in hormone levels, including increases in cortisol and decreases in insulin, can impact sleep quality. These hormonal adjustments may cause variations in sleep architecture, the pattern of sleep cycles including deep, light, and REM sleep, potentially leading to difficulties in falling and staying asleep.

Optimising your fasting regimen to support better sleep involves careful timing of your eating and fasting periods.

Consuming your last meal a few hours before bedtime can prevent sleep disturbances linked to digestion and metabolism. Specifically, avoiding heavy, rich meals or foods that are high in sugar close to bedtime can help prevent spikes in blood sugar levels, which can keep you awake. Additionally, steering clear of caffeine late in the day is advisable as it can significantly impair your ability to fall asleep. Caffeine blocks the adenosine receptors in your brain, which are responsible for making you feel sleepy, thereby delaying your sleep cycle. Establishing a consistent eating schedule that aligns with your circadian rhythms - eating during daylight hours and fasting through the night - can further enhance sleep quality by syncing your metabolic processes with your body's natural biological clock.

Supplements can also play a supportive role in enhancing sleep, especially when your body is adjusting to a new fasting schedule. Natural supplements like melatonin, known as the sleep hormone, can be particularly beneficial. Melatonin levels naturally rise in the evening to promote sleep and decrease in the morning to help wake you up. If you find that fasting temporarily disrupts this natural cycle, a melatonin supplement might help recalibrate your internal clock. Another useful supplement is magnesium, which plays a role in supporting deep, restorative sleep by maintaining healthy levels of GABA, a neurotransmitter that promotes sleep. Magnesium's relaxation effect on the nervous system can help improve sleep quality and make it easier to fall asleep. It's important to consult with a healthcare provider before starting any supplement, particularly to ensure they do not interfere with other medications you may be taking and to establish the correct dosage.

Creating a restful environment is equally important for good sleep hygiene. This can be achieved by reducing exposure to blue light emitted by screens such as televisions, smartphones, and computers, which can suppress the natural production of melatonin and disrupt your sleep cycle. Consider setting a digital curfew an hour or so before bed, replacing screen time with relaxing activities such as reading a book, listening to soothing music, or practising relaxation exercises like deep breathing or gentle yoga. Additionally, maintaining a regular sleep schedule - going to bed and waking up at the same time every day, including weekends - can help regulate your body's sleep-wake cycle, making it easier to fall asleep and wake up naturally.

By understanding the link between fasting, hormone regulation, and sleep, and implementing strategies to align these elements harmoniously, you can enhance not only the quality of your sleep but also the effectiveness of your fasting regimen. This holistic approach supports your body's natural rhythms, promoting restorative sleep that rejuvenates and prepares you for the day ahead, ensuring that you can fully enjoy the benefits of your intermittent fasting lifestyle.

Boosting Energy Levels through Targeted Fasting

One of the marvellous adaptations of the human body is its ability to adjust its energy management systems in response to dietary intake, and intermittent fasting plays a pivotal role in this adjustment. Initially, you might experience a dip in your energy levels as your body shifts from relying primarily on glucose to a more balanced use of fat as fuel. This transition period is critical and understanding it can help mitigate discomfort and optimise energy use. As your body becomes accustomed to intermittent fasting, it increases its metabolic flexibility, which is the ability to efficiently switch between using carbs and fats for energy. This not only stabilises your energy levels but also improves overall energy efficiency, reducing feelings of lethargy and fatigue. Good fat such as olive oil, coconut oil, egg yolks and fatty fish are necessary for hormone production including testosterone levels which keep us from losing energy and libido.

To make the most of your eating windows and sustain your energy throughout fasting periods, strategic nutrition is key. Incorporating foods rich in complex carbohydrates, such as legumes, and vegetables, provides a slow and steady release of glucose, which helps maintain steady energy levels. These foods are also rich in fibre, which slows down digestion and prolongs the feeling of fullness. Healthy fats, found in foods like avocados, nuts, seeds, and olive oil, are also essential. They not only provide a dense energy source but also support cell function and hormonal balance, which can be particularly beneficial during menopause. Combining these nutrients effectively can help you manage your energy efficiently, making fasting and eating periods more manageable and productive.

During fasting periods, it's not uncommon to experience energy slumps, especially in the early stages of adapting to the fasting lifestyle. One practical way to manage these slumps is through short, light physical activities such as walking or stretching. These activities stimulate blood flow and increase energy levels without requiring a significant caloric expenditure. Strategic hydration is also crucial; dehydration can often masquerade as fatigue. Ensuring you drink adequate fluids, especially water, can help maintain energy levels and aid in overall metabolism and detoxification processes during fasting.

The long-term benefits of intermittent fasting on energy are profound. One significant benefit is the improvement of mitochondrial function. Mitochondria are often referred to as the powerhouses of the cells; they generate the energy that our cells need to function. Fasting has been shown to stimulate mitochondrial biogenesis, the process by which new mitochondria are formed within the cells. This not only enhances the cells' energy-producing capabilities but also plays a role in ageing and longevity. Additionally, intermittent fasting reduces oxidative stress and inflammation, two factors that can sap energy and cause cellular damage. By reducing these, your body can function more efficiently, and you feel more energised and capable of handling your daily activities.

By understanding these aspects of how intermittent fasting can influence and enhance your energy levels, you're better equipped to optimise your fasting and eating schedules to support your energy throughout the day. This proactive approach allows you to enjoy the benefits of intermittent fasting without compromising your vitality, enabling you to engage fully in your daily life and activities.

As this chapter concludes, we've explored a variety of strategies to enhance your experience with intermittent fasting, particularly through the lens of managing and optimising energy levels. From understanding the initial impacts of fasting on your body's energy management to implementing dietary strategies and physical activities that support sustained energy, these insights are designed to empower you with the knowledge to make intermittent fasting a beneficial part of your lifestyle. As we continue on, the focus will shift to further integrating intermittent fasting into your life, ensuring that it complements your health goals and supports your journey towards wellness.

Chapter 4

Overcoming Challenges & Handling Setbacks

When embarking on the path of intermittent fasting, it's akin to navigating a new terrain that promises lush landscapes but requires crossing a few streams and climbing some steep slopes. You may have set out on this journey filled with enthusiasm, only to find yourself facing the challenge of managing hunger. It's a common hurdle, yet how you handle this can define your experience and success with intermittent fasting. Drawing from my own expedition through the rugged terrains of dietary changes, I've gathered insights and strategies to help you manage hunger effectively, maintaining your course towards a healthier lifestyle without feeling overwhelmed by temporary obstacles.

Coping with Hunger: Practical Tips & Tricks

Understanding Hunger Signals

The first step in mastering hunger during intermittent fasting is differentiating between true hunger and habitual eating cues. True hunger is your body's natural signal that it needs fuel, characterised by physical cues like a growling stomach, low energy, and even slight irritability, colloquially known as being 'hangry'. In contrast, habitual eating cues are often triggered by environmental factors, emotions, or specific times of the day - like reaching for a snack during your favourite TV show out of routine rather than need.

To navigate this, start by tuning into your body's signals. Before reaching for food, pause and ask yourself if you are truly hungry or if you're responding to a habit or emotion. This simple pause can help you start to break the cycle of non-hungry eating and make more mindful decisions about when to eat. A cup of green tea with a dash of apple cider vinegar is my go to remedy and it is well researched as an appetite suppressant.

Mindful Eating Techniques

When you do eat, practising mindful eating can transform your relationship with food. Mindful eating involves paying full attention to the experience of eating and drinking, both inside and outside the body. Notice the colours, smells, textures, and flavours of your food, and chew slowly, savouring each bite. Eating in this deliberate manner can enhance your appreciation of meals, reduce overeating, and increase satiety.

A practical way to integrate mindful eating into your routine is by setting down your utensils between bites or taking a sip of water, which naturally slows down your meal and helps you assess your fullness levels more accurately. This practice not only helps in managing portion sizes but also enhances digestion and satisfaction with smaller meals, which is particularly beneficial during the eating windows in intermittent fasting.

Hunger Management Strategies

Effective hunger management is pivotal in maintaining your fasting schedule without discomfort. One effective strategy is to drink plenty of water throughout the day. Dehydration often masquerades as hunger, so keeping hydrated can stave off unwarranted hunger pangs.

Additionally, consider incorporating low-calorie beverages like herbal teas or bone broth during your fasting periods. These can help fill the void without breaking your fast, providing comfort and a sense of fullness.

Another useful technique is engaging in light activities to distract from hunger. During fasting periods, if you find yourself fixated on thoughts of food, try redirecting your attention to activities such as walking, light stretching, or any hobby that keeps your hands and mind busy. This not only helps you navigate through the fasting period more comfortably but also enriches your day with fulfilling and engaging tasks.

Nutrient-Dense Foods for Satiety

When you do eat, choosing the right foods can significantly impact how full you feel. Focus on incorporating foods that are high in fibre, protein, and healthy fats, all of which are known for their satiating properties. Foods like avocados, legumes, free range meats, and nuts not only keep you fuller for longer but also provide the nutrients needed to support your health during fasting.

For instance, starting your eating window with a salad loaded with leafy greens, seeds, and a portion of grilled chicken or tofu can provide a high-fibre, high-protein meal that keeps satiety high. Ending your eating window with a snack rich in healthy fats, such as a handful of almonds or a small natural unsweetened yoghurt, can help maintain a feeling of fullness as you enter your fasting period.

By understanding and implementing these strategies, you can effectively manage hunger during intermittent fasting, turning what might seem like a daunting challenge into a manageable part of your health journey. These practices not only aid in adhering to your fasting schedule but also enhance your overall relationship with food, leading to a healthier, more mindful approach to eating. As you continue to apply these tips and tricks, remember that each step forward, no matter how small, is a progress towards mastering your body's cues and optimising your fasting experience.

How to Handle Social Eating & Holidays

Navigating social eating and holiday feasts while maintaining an intermittent fasting schedule might seem daunting at first glance. You might worry about sticking to your eating plan without feeling left out of the festive indulgences or family dinners. However, with a few strategic approaches, you can enjoy these gatherings without compromising your fasting routine, ensuring that your social life and dietary goals harmoniously coexist.

Firstly, planning ahead is crucial when you know you'll be attending a social event. This doesn't just mean marking the event on your calendar; it involves planning your fasting and eating windows around the event. If you're on a 16/8 intermittent fasting schedule and a dinner party is set for the evening, consider shifting your eating window to later in the day so it aligns with the event. This way, you can partake in the meal without having to explain why you're not eating or feeling like you're missing out. Before the event, review the menu if available, or if you're dining at someone's home, don't hesitate to ask what will be served. This can help you anticipate your options and make choices that align with your nutritional goals. For instance, knowing that grilled salmon, a rich source of protein and omega-3 fatty acids, will be served can reassure you that you can maintain a balanced diet during the event.

Communicating your dietary preferences effectively to hosts or dining companions is another important aspect of navigating social eating. There's often a concern about coming off as rude or high-maintenance, but most friends and family are accommodating once they understand your goals. Explain that you are following an intermittent fasting plan, which has specific eating times for health reasons. Most people will respect your choices and might even take interest in learning more about them. It's helpful to focus on the positive aspects - emphasise that this schedule makes you feel great and is part of your commitment to maintaining your health. Offering to bring a dish that fits your eating plan can also be a discreet and generous way to ensure there's something suitable for you to eat without imposing your dietary choices on others.

Embracing flexible fasting strategies can also reduce stress around social eating. If an event falls outside your usual eating window, giving yourself permission to adjust for that day can help maintain the enjoyment of social interactions. For example, if you typically finish eating by 6pm but a friend's birthday dinner is at 7 pm, it's perfectly acceptable to adapt for this occasion. Flexibility is key in making intermittent fasting a sustainable lifestyle choice rather than a restrictive diet. Just remember to return to your regular fasting schedule the following day. This adaptability can prevent feelings of guilt and help you balance your social life with your health goals.

Lastly, making mindful choices at these events can empower you to enjoy yourself without overindulgence. Focus on foods that are both satisfying and nourishing. Fill your plate with vegetables, lean proteins, and healthy fats, and savour each bite. This not only aligns with your fasting goals but also enhances your overall enjoyment of the meal. If faced with a buffet, take a moment to survey all the options before making your selections, and avoid going back for second helpings immediately. If you decide to indulge in a dessert or a special dish, do so consciously, enjoying the flavours and the experience rather than eating out of habit.

By approaching social eating and holidays with a plan, communicating your needs effectively, allowing flexibility in your fasting schedule, and making mindful food choices, you can navigate these challenges with ease and confidence. This balanced approach ensures that you can enjoy the social and celebratory aspects of dining with friends and family while staying committed to your intermittent fasting lifestyle.

Adjusting your Fasting Plan as you Age

As time gracefully unfolds, our bodies undergo a symphony of changes, each note resonating with our evolving needs and capacities. Embracing these changes, especially as we venture deeper into our 50s and beyond, necessitates a thoughtful recalibration of our intermittent fasting strategies. Regular health assessments become pivotal during this period. These check-ups are not just routine appointments;

they are insightful sessions where you can discuss your fasting regimen with healthcare professionals who understand the nuances of ageing. These assessments can help tailor your fasting plan to better suit your metabolic needs, which inevitably shift as you age. For instance, if your doctor notices changes in your blood glucose levels or blood pressure, modifications to your fasting schedule or dietary intake might be recommended to optimise your health outcomes. If your doctor is unfamiliar with intermittent fasting you can find another or refer him to the work of Dr. Michael Mosely so sadly recently deceased, for the UK, Dr. Jason Fung in Canada and the US or Dr. Oz who has regular TV appearances in the US. All of them recognise the huge benefits of fasting.

Listening to your body's signals plays a critical role in this adaptive process. This attunement goes beyond mere observation; it involves an active engagement with your body's cues. For example, if you find that longer fasting periods leave you feeling unusually fatigued or irritable, it might be a sign to shorten the fasting window. Conversely, you might discover that you feel energised and mentally clear with a slightly extended fast, suggesting that your body can handle and perhaps benefit from a longer fasting duration. The key is to adjust these lengths and frequencies not arbitrarily, but based on careful listening to your body's responses. This approach ensures that your fasting regimen supports your well-being without compromising your comfort or health.

Adapting to physical changes with age is another crucial consideration. As we age, our body's tolerance for fasting can change. Metabolic rate slows, muscle mass naturally decreases, and digestive efficiency might not be what it once was. These changes require a flexible approach to fasting - one that respects our body's evolving capabilities. For instance, if muscle preservation becomes a concern, focusing your eating windows on protein-rich meals can help counteract muscle loss, and adjusting fasting times to include a post-exercise meal can optimise muscle recovery and growth. Similarly, if digestive issues arise, adjusting meal timing to earlier in the day when digestive capabilities are stronger might be beneficial.

Incorporating preventative nutrition into your eating windows is essential to support your changing body's needs. Nutrient-dense foods that bolster bone health, muscle mass, and cognitive function should be cornerstones of your diet. Calcium-rich foods like dairy or fortified alternatives, and vitamin D, either through exposure to sunlight or supplements, are crucial for maintaining bone density. Omega-3 fatty acids, found in fish like salmon and in flaxseeds, support brain health and can help maintain muscle mass. Antioxidant-rich foods like berries and dark leafy greens can combat oxidative stress, a key factor in ageing. Planning your meals to include these nutrients can help not only in managing the physical aspects of ageing but also in enhancing your overall vitality.

As you continue to adapt your fasting strategy with age, remember that these adjustments are not about clinging to youth but about embracing your maturity with a strategy that brings out the best in your health. This adaptive approach allows you to continue enjoying the benefits of intermittent fasting, tailored to your body's current needs, ensuring that your later years are lived with vigour and wellness.

Dealing with Plateaus: Advanced Strategies

When you initially embrace intermittent fasting, it's common to see noticeable results quite quickly - whether it's weight loss, improved energy, or better metabolic health. However, over time, you might find yourself facing a plateau where progress seems to stall. This can be particularly frustrating, especially when you feel you're doing everything 'right'.

Understanding why these plateaus occur, especially in the context of ageing and hormonal changes, is the first step in moving past them.

Weight loss plateaus are often a natural part of the weight loss process, but for women over 50, they can also be compounded by hormonal fluctuations and changes in body composition. As oestrogen levels decline during menopause, your body tends to hold onto fat more stubbornly, particularly around the abdomen, as a physiological response to lower hormone levels. Additionally, as we age, our basal metabolic rate (the amount of energy expended while at rest) decreases. This means that even if you continue eating the same amount of calories that used to help you lose weight, it might now only be enough to maintain your weight. Recognizing this shift is crucial in adjusting your approach to continue seeing results. Let the fasting be your way to lower calorie intake and lower your carbohydrates and increase fats as on the ketogenic diet. This should avoid calorie counting and increase energy, motivation and satiety.

To intensify your fasting windows safely, consider gradually extending your fasting periods. If you've been comfortable with a 16/8 fasting plan, extending to an 18/6 plan could renew progress. This adjustment increases the duration your body spends in the fat-burning phase, potentially shaking off the plateau. For those who are more experienced and medically cleared by their healthcare providers, incorporating an occasional 24-hour fast can provide a metabolic reset, boosting growth hormone levels and further enhancing fat oxidation. However, these adjustments should be made gradually and with consideration of how your body responds. It's important to ensure that any intensification of your fasting regimen still allows you to consume adequate nutrients during your eating windows.

Cross-training and resistance exercises are another effective strategy to counteract weight loss plateaus. While intermittent fasting helps to manage calorie intake, exercise increases calorie expenditure, creating a more significant energy deficit. Cross-training, which involves alternating different types of exercise (such as cycling, swimming, and running), prevents your body from adapting too much to one activity, keeping your metabolism active and engaged. Resistance training, such as weight lifting or using resistance bands, is particularly beneficial as it helps build and preserve lean muscle mass. Since muscle tissue burns more calories than fat tissue, increasing your muscle mass can help boost your metabolic rate, making it easier to overcome a weight loss plateau.

Incorporating these exercises into your routine not only aids in breaking through plateaus but also supports healthy ageing by improving bone density, enhancing flexibility, and reducing the risk of chronic diseases.

By adopting these advanced strategies, you can better manage and move past plateaus in your weight loss journey. Whether it's reassessing caloric needs, adjusting fasting lengths, or incorporating varied physical activities, each adjustment is a stepping stone towards revitalising your progress and pushing towards your health goals. Remember, the key to successful intermittent fasting, especially as you age, lies in the ability to adapt and fine-tune your approach based on your body's evolving needs.

When to Break a Fast Safely & Healthily

Embarking on an intermittent fasting regimen introduces you to the nuances of your body's responses in ways you might not have noticed before. It's a process that demands not just commitment but also an acute awareness of how your body reacts under different conditions. Recognizing the signs that necessitate ending a fast early is crucial, not only to prevent adverse effects but to ensure that fasting remains a beneficial and sustainable practice.

Significant fatigue, dizziness, and cognitive impairment are clear indicators that your body might not be coping well with the fasting regime at that moment. These symptoms can arise from various factors, such as inadequate hydration, insufficient nutrient intake during eating windows, or more serious underlying health issues. If you experience severe or persistent symptoms, it is wise to listen to your body and end the fast early. This isn't a setback but rather a necessary step in managing your health responsibly.

Breaking a fast safely involves reintroducing food in a way that doesn't overwhelm your digestive system. After a period of not eating, your digestive enzymes and hormones that manage food intake need to readjust. Starting with light, easily digestible foods can prevent any gastrointestinal discomfort and help your body better assimilate nutrients.

A small meal that includes components like cooked vegetables, broth, yoghurt, or bone broth is ideal. These foods are gentle on the stomach and provide a balanced mix of proteins, and fats, which help stabilise blood sugar levels gradually without causing a significant insulin spike. It's also beneficial to continue hydrating with water or an electrolyte-rich drink to support the digestive process and replenish any fluids lost during the fast.

Listening to your body's health signals is an integral part of practising intermittent fasting, especially as you navigate the varying needs of your system. This might mean altering your fasting schedule based on how you feel on a particular day or over a period. For instance, if you consistently notice signs of hypoglycemia, such as shaking, sweating, or intense hunger, during longer fasts, it may be necessary to shorten your fasting periods or adjust the timing of your meals to accommodate your body's glucose requirements. Similarly, if digestive issues occur frequently when breaking your fast, it might indicate the need for a more gradual refeeding or that certain foods need to be reintroduced more slowly to assess tolerance.

In navigating the complexities of intermittent fasting, especially for women over 50, understanding when and how to safely break a fast is as important as managing the fasting periods themselves. This knowledge empowers you to make informed decisions that enhance your wellbeing and ensure that intermittent fasting remains a positive and healthful part of your lifestyle.

Emotional Eating & Fasting: Finding Balance

The intertwining of emotions and eating is a complex dance that many of us find ourselves engaged in, often without conscious thought. Particularly during periods like menopause, when hormonal fluctuations are at their peak, you might find yourself reaching for comfort foods as a way to manage stress, sadness, or even joy. Recognizing when your eating habits are driven by emotions rather than physical hunger is a crucial step in maintaining not only your fasting regimen but also in fostering a healthier relationship with food.

Identifying triggers for emotional eating can be quite revealing. These triggers can be anything from a stressful day at work, a fight with a loved friend, boredom, or even the ambiance of a cosy, rainy afternoon. When fasting, these triggers might feel more pronounced due to the heightened awareness of your eating habits. Taking the time to understand what prompts your emotional eating helps in developing strategies to manage it. Keeping a food and mood diary can be an effective way to track these moments. Note what you eat, when, and what you're feeling at the time. Over time, patterns will likely emerge, providing insights into which emotions are likely to send you to the kitchen.

Developing strategies to manage emotional eating involves finding alternatives to eating that still address your emotional needs. For example, if you find that stress drives you to snack, consider whether activities like journaling could serve as an outlet for your stress instead. Writing down your thoughts and feelings can be incredibly cathartic and a way to deal with emotions productively. If loneliness sends you searching for comfort food, picking up the phone and talking to a friend or joining a social group can help fulfil your need for connection. Engaging in hobbies that keep your hands and mind busy, such as knitting, painting, or gardening, can also redirect your focus from food to tasks that bring satisfaction and joy.

Incorporating relaxation techniques into your routine can also play a significant role in managing the emotional urges to eat. Techniques such as deep breathing, yoga, or meditation can reduce stress and enhance your overall emotional balance, making you less likely to turn to food for emotional comfort. Deep breathing exercises, for example, can be done almost anywhere and require only a few minutes to ground your thoughts and ease stress. Yoga combines physical postures, breathing exercises, and meditation, helping to release tension and improve mood.

Regular practice can offer a refuge from the daily triggers of emotional eating, providing a nurturing space for your body and mind.

Balancing emotional well-being is a critical component of a successful fasting plan. It's important to recognize that addressing emotional eating is not just about controlling food intake; it's about understanding and managing your emotional health, which is just as vital as your physical health. This holistic approach ensures that your fasting journey is not only about nourishing your body but also about caring for your emotional and mental well-being. By acknowledging and addressing the emotional aspects of eating, you enhance your ability to maintain your fasting regimen effectively, supporting your overall health and happiness.

As we wrap up this chapter on overcoming challenges and handling setbacks, we've explored various strategies that support your fasting journey - from managing hunger and navigating social settings to adjusting your fasting plan as you age and dealing with emotional eating. Each section has equipped you with practical tools and insights to not only face these challenges but to embrace them as opportunities for growth and learning in your fasting journey.

As we move forward, the focus will shift to integrating intermittent fasting into your life in a way that feels natural and sustainable, ensuring that this practice enhances your health and complements your lifestyle.

Chapter 5

Integrating Intermittent Fasting with Overall Wellness

Imagine you're standing at the edge of a serene lake, the surface so smooth it mirrors the vast, unblemished sky above. Dipping your toes into the water, you expect a shock of cold, but instead, you're greeted by a surprising warmth, inviting you to wade deeper. This feeling, unexpected yet profoundly right, is akin to discovering the psychological and cognitive benefits of intermittent fasting - a journey that not only transforms your body but also elevates your mind and spirit.

The Psychological Benefits of Intermittent Fasting

Enhanced Mental Clarity & Focus

One of the most celebrated effects of intermittent fasting is the remarkable improvement in mental clarity and focus many experience. This isn't just anecdotal; science supports it too. During fasting, your body undergoes a metabolic shift from using glucose to fatty acids and ketones for energy. This shift not only promotes a more stable energy supply but reduces inflammation, a known disruptor of cognitive processes. Moreover, intermittent fasting increases the levels of brain-derived neurotrophic factor (BDNF), a protein that plays a key role in neuron growth and the maintenance of brain health. BDNF is often likened to fertiliser for the brain - it helps brain cells thrive and connect, which is crucial for learning and memory. Research published in the Journal of Neurochemistry found that fasting can lead to an increase in BDNF, linking it to improved brain function and resilience against stress-related disorders.

Mood Improvement

The impact of intermittent fasting on mood is profound and multifaceted. Fluctuations in blood sugar levels can send your emotions on a rollercoaster ride, with spikes and dips that can leave you feeling irritable or anxious. Intermittent fasting helps to stabilise these levels, leading to improved mood stability. Additionally, the ketones produced during fasting have been shown to have a mood-stabilising effect.

A study published in the Archives of General Psychiatry observed that ketones could help mitigate symptoms of depression and bipolar disorder. The exact mechanisms are still being studied, but the anti-inflammatory effects of ketones and their role in fueling brain function are believed to be significant factors.

Increased Resilience to Stress

Fasting teaches your body and mind to endure and adapt to stress, which enhances your overall resilience. This adaptive response is known as hormesis, a process where moderate stress stimulates the body to improve its stress resistance. This can be particularly empowering for women over 50, who often juggle multiple roles and responsibilities. The discipline of maintaining a fasting schedule, and the self-control it requires, builds mental and emotional strength, making you better equipped to handle life's challenges. Furthermore, the physiological benefits of fasting, such as improved metabolic health and reduced inflammation, support a more balanced and less reactive stress response system.

Long-Term Cognitive Benefits

Perhaps one of the most compelling reasons to integrate intermittent fasting into your lifestyle is its potential to protect against neurodegenerative diseases. Studies suggest that the metabolic and cellular benefits of fasting - such as reduced oxidative stress and enhanced cellular cleanup processes - may lower the risk of diseases like Alzheimer's and Parkinson's. A study in the New England Journal of Medicine highlighted intermittent fasting's role in increasing neuronal resistance to genetic and environmental factors that typically precede such diseases. While more research is needed, the potential of intermittent fasting to contribute to a healthier, more agile brain as you age is an exciting prospect.

Embracing intermittent fasting can feel like wading into uncharted waters, but as you acclimate, you'll find it can be as refreshing and invigorating as that warm lake on a serene day.

The mental clarity, mood stability, resilience, and cognitive benefits are not just promises; they are profound changes that can redefine your health trajectory. As you continue to explore the integration of intermittent fasting into your life, consider these psychological and cognitive enhancements as key motivators that underscore the holistic benefits of this life-changing practice.

Mindful Eating Practices During Your Eating Window

In the bustling rhythm of daily life, meals often become just another task on our checklist, something we do while multitasking, whether it's catching up on emails or watching the evening news. Yet, what if I told you that changing the way you eat could transform the way you feel during your eating window and beyond? Mindful eating, a practice rooted in ancient traditions, invites you to experience eating as a nourishing ritual rather than a rushed necessity. At its core, mindful eating is about engaging fully with the experience of eating, focusing on each bite, and noticing the flavours, textures, and effects on your body without distraction. This practice not only enhances your relationship with food but also aligns beautifully with intermittent fasting, where every meal is an opportunity to nourish and satiate your body effectively.

Imagine sitting down to your first meal after a fasting period; instead of hastily consuming your food, you take a moment to really look at what's on your plate, appreciating the colours and aromas. You take a slow bite, chewing thoroughly, which is the first step in digestion and an excellent practice to aid nutrient absorption. Chewing slowly allows the digestive enzymes in your saliva to start breaking down food, making it easier to digest and ensuring you extract maximum nutrients. This practice also helps regulate your eating pace, which can lead to better digestion and a more satisfying meal. Additionally, by avoiding distractions such as electronic devices during meals, you can tune into your body's hunger and fullness signals more effectively. This can prevent overeating, which is common when we eat absentmindedly, and helps maintain a healthy weight - crucial for post-menopausal women who often struggle with weight gain due to hormonal changes.

The benefits of mindful eating extend beyond the physical. When you eat mindfully, you're likely to find that meals become more satisfying, and you may need less food to feel full.

This is particularly beneficial during your eating window in intermittent fasting, as it can prevent the tendency to overeat after a period of fasting. Feeling more satisfied with smaller portions can help maintain a healthy caloric intake and lead to long-term weight management.

Improved digestion is another significant benefit. By eating slowly and chewing thoroughly, you reduce the digestive system's workload and decrease issues like bloating and gas, which are not uncommon when large meals are consumed quickly.

Incorporating mindfulness into your eating doesn't have to stop when you leave the table. Extending these practices into other areas of your life, such as mindful walking or meditation, can amplify the benefits of intermittent fasting by enhancing your overall well-being. Taking a mindful walk, where you focus on your breath and the sensations of your feet touching the ground, can be a wonderful way to connect with nature and clear your mind, reducing stress levels. Meditation, even if practised for just a few minutes a day, can improve your stress management, enhance your focus, and stabilise your mood. These practices can help cultivate a state of mindfulness that benefits all areas of your life, leading to a more balanced, health-focused approach to your daily routine.

By embracing mindful eating and extending mindfulness to other aspects of your life, you not only enhance your intermittent fasting experience but also foster a deeper connection to your body's needs and responses.

This holistic approach can transform your eating window from a routine part of your day into a rejuvenating practice that nourishes both your body and mind, setting a strong foundation for lasting health and wellness. As you continue to explore and integrate these practices, you may find that the benefits extend far beyond your meals, enriching your overall experience of life and well-being.

Low-Impact Exercises That Complement Fasting

Integrating exercise into your intermittent fasting routine can seem like a delicate balancing act, especially when you're trying to match your workout times with your eating and fasting windows. However, low-impact exercises such as swimming, cycling, and yoga not only offer a fantastic synergy with fasting but are also particularly well-suited for women over 50. These activities provide adequate physical stimulus to keep you fit and active without the strenuous impact on your joints and muscles that more intense exercises might entail.

Swimming, for instance, is a wonderful whole-body exercise that enhances cardiovascular health while being easy on the joints. It's an ideal activity for those who might be dealing with arthritis or other joint issues that can become more prevalent as you age. Cycling, whether outdoors or on a stationary bike, is another excellent low-impact exercise that strengthens your legs and improves heart health without harsh impact on your hips, knees, and ankles. Yoga, known for its flexibility and balance benefits, not only supports physical health but also incorporates elements of meditation that can enhance mental focus and reduce stress, making it a holistic practice beneficial to both body and mind.

Timing your exercise in relation to your fasting schedule can significantly affect how you feel during your workout and how your body uses fuel. Engaging in low-impact exercise just before your eating window opens can be particularly effective. This timing takes advantage of your body's shift towards burning fat for fuel, which occurs after longer periods of fasting. Exercising during this time can increase fat burn and, immediately following your workout with your first meal can help your body replenish and recover more efficiently. For instance, a morning yoga session that ends as your eating window begins can allow you to immediately follow up with a protein-rich breakfast to aid muscle recovery and hydration.

The benefits of incorporating regular low-impact exercise into your routine extend far beyond immediate energy expenditure. Regular physical activity is crucial for maintaining cardiovascular health, which is especially important as heart disease risks increase with age.

Exercise also plays a significant role in improving flexibility and balance, which can help prevent falls - a common concern for ageing adults. Moreover, maintaining muscle mass through activities like cycling and swimming can combat the natural muscle degradation that occurs with ageing, helping you maintain a healthier metabolism and better overall physical function.

Personalising your exercise routine is key to making it enjoyable and sustainable. Start by assessing your current fitness level and any physical limitations you might have. Consider what times of day you feel most energetic and how these times align with your fasting schedule. If you prefer starting your day with activity, morning exercises before your first meal can invigorate your day and optimise fat burning. If you find you have more energy later in the day, scheduling a swim or a bike ride before your evening meal can help you wind down and ensure you're replenishing your body post-exercise. It's also important to vary your activities to keep your routine interesting and cover different aspects of fitness. For example, you might combine yoga on one day to improve flexibility and balance, with cycling on another to enhance cardiovascular health and leg strength. This variety not only keeps your routine engaging but also ensures a more comprehensive approach to fitness, addressing different physical needs and preventing overuse injuries.

As you integrate these low-impact exercises into your lifestyle, remember to listen to your body and adjust your activities as needed. What works well one month might need adjustment the next as your body changes or as you find what types of exercise you most enjoy. The goal is to find a routine that feels good, fits your lifestyle, and complements your intermittent fasting schedule, helping you maintain an active, fulfilling lifestyle.

Hydration & its Crucial Role in Fasting

Understanding the importance of staying hydrated, especially during fasting periods, is akin to recognizing the need for water in a flourishing garden. Just as plants wilt without adequate moisture, your body, too, can't function optimally without proper hydration. During fasting, every cell and system in your body still requires water to carry out essential metabolic processes.

Water helps to metabolise and transport nutrients, regulate body temperature, and detoxify your body by removing waste products. Moreover, hydration plays a pivotal role in managing hunger - often, feelings of hunger are actually signs of dehydration. By staying well-hydrated, you can more accurately assess your hunger levels, which is crucial for maintaining effective fasting periods without giving into unnecessary snacking that can derail your progress.

But hydration during fasting isn't just about drinking plain water. Exploring hydration sources beyond water, such as herbal teas and infused waters, can enhance your fasting experience, adding variety and additional health benefits. Herbal teas, for example, are wonderful companions during fasting. They not only provide hydration without calories but can also offer soothing and digestive benefits. Peppermint tea, with its natural muscle relaxant properties, can help alleviate digestive issues like bloating and spasms. Ginger tea stimulates digestion and boosts metabolism, making it a warming and beneficial drink during colder days or when you need a metabolic lift. Infused waters, another delightful option, make hydration more enjoyable. Adding slices of fruits like lemon, lime, or cucumber, or herbs like mint or basil, can transform a simple glass of water into a refreshing and flavorful treat that encourages more frequent sipping.

Monitoring your hydration status is crucial, especially as you adapt to an intermittent fasting schedule. Recognizing signs of dehydration is key to preventing it before it impacts your health. Common signs include headaches, dizziness, dry mouth, dark-coloured urine, and fatigue. These symptoms can affect your concentration and physical performance, making daily tasks and especially any form of exercise more challenging. To monitor your hydration status effectively, pay attention to the colour of your urine.

A light straw colour indicates good hydration, while darker shades suggest a need for increased fluid intake. Keeping a hydration tracker or using a mobile app can also help you stay on top of your water intake by sending reminders to drink water throughout the day, ensuring you meet your hydration needs consistently.

To improve your water intake, integration into your daily routine is essential. Setting reminders on your phone or keeping a visible water bottle with you throughout the day can serve as constant cues to drink water. You might also consider starting your day with a large glass of water to kickstart hydration early, setting a positive tone for the rest of the day. Additionally, incorporating water-rich foods into your meals can significantly boost hydration.

Foods like cucumbers and celery contain high amounts of water and the added benefit of fibre, vitamins, and minerals. These strategies not only help maintain adequate hydration but also support your overall health and enhance the effectiveness of your fasting regimen.

Stress Management Techniques for Better Fasting Results

Understanding how stress influences our eating habits is crucial, especially when integrating intermittent fasting into your lifestyle. Stress, particularly chronic stress, can significantly derail your fasting efforts, leading to impulsive eating behaviours and choices that are not aligned with your health goals. During stressful times, the body releases cortisol, a hormone that can increase appetite and cravings for high-calorie foods. This biological response was useful in our evolutionary past when stress often indicated a need for extra energy for fight-or-flight situations. However, in today's world, chronic stress can lead to prolonged cortisol elevations which may sabotage your fasting and dietary intentions by compelling you to reach for comfort foods during your eating windows or even outside them.

To counteract the effects of stress on your eating habits, incorporating effective stress-reduction techniques into both your fasting and non-fasting periods is essential. Progressive muscle relaxation (PMR) is a method that involves tensing each muscle group in your body intensely, but briefly, and then suddenly releasing the tension. This exercise helps in reducing physical and mental tension. Practising PMR can be particularly beneficial during your fasting periods when you might feel more susceptible to stress. By relieving physical tension, PMR can help diminish overall stress levels, making it easier to adhere to your fasting schedule without succumbing to stress-induced eating.

Deep breathing exercises offer another potent tool in managing stress. Techniques such as diaphragmatic breathing involve focusing on deep, even breaths that engage the diaphragm, helping to slow your heartbeat and lower blood pressure, creating a sense of calm that can aid in managing stress-induced urges to eat. Setting aside time for deep breathing during your fasting periods can help maintain a calm and focused mind, essential for sustaining your fasting regimen.

Guided imagery, another effective stress-reduction technique, involves visualising a peaceful scene or scenario to divert your mind from current stressors. This technique can be particularly useful during fasting when thoughts of food might be more prevalent. By mentally transporting yourself to a serene environment, your body can experience a relaxation response similar to what happens when you are actually in a calming environment, helping decrease the urge to engage in stress-eating.

Integrating these stress management techniques into your daily life can enhance the effectiveness of intermittent fasting and your overall well-being. Establish a routine that includes dedicated time for these practices, perhaps in the morning to set a positive tone for the day or during your fasting periods when you might need stress relief the most. Consistency is key in reaping the benefits; just as intermittent fasting requires a schedule, effective stress management is most beneficial when practised regularly.

The role of adequate sleep in managing stress and supporting your fasting efforts cannot be overstated. Sleep and stress have a bidirectional relationship - just as poor sleep can increase stress levels, high stress can lead to sleep disturbances. Good sleep hygiene, which includes habits and practices that are conducive to sleeping well on a regular basis, is vital. This includes maintaining a consistent sleep schedule, creating a restful sleeping environment, and avoiding stimulants like caffeine close to bedtime. Prioritising good sleep hygiene can improve the quality of your sleep, thus reducing stress and making it easier to maintain your fasting schedule. Adequate sleep supports hormonal balance, including the regulation of ghrelin and leptin, hormones that control hunger and satiety, which are crucial for successful intermittent fasting.

By adopting these stress management techniques and prioritising good sleep hygiene, you can create a supportive environment for your fasting regime, enabling you to manage stress effectively and maintain your commitment to your health goals. This proactive approach not only enhances your ability to stick to intermittent fasting but also contributes to a healthier, more balanced lifestyle.

Building a Support Network for Fasting Success

One of the most enriching aspects of embracing intermittent fasting is the sense of community and support that can arise from sharing this journey. Whether you're discussing your fasting schedule over coffee with a friend or exchanging recipes in an online forum, the benefits of having a support network are immense.

These connections provide not only emotional encouragement but also practical tips and shared experiences that can make your fasting journey smoother and more enjoyable.

Imagine having a group of friends or an online community where you can share your successes and seek advice during challenging times. This network becomes a resource, offering insights into what works and what doesn't, which can be especially valuable when you're adjusting to a new eating pattern or overcoming a plateau. The emotional support from others who understand exactly what you're going through can be incredibly motivating. It's comforting to know you're not alone in your efforts to improve your health. This sense of shared endeavour can make all the difference in maintaining your motivation and commitment.

Finding these communities might seem daunting, but there are numerous ways to connect with like-minded individuals. Online, numerous forums and social media groups are dedicated to intermittent fasting. These platforms are fantastic resources where you can ask questions, share your experiences, and learn from others' insights. Websites like Reddit offer subreddits related to fasting where thousands of members regularly discuss their routines and challenges. Similarly, Facebook has many groups for intermittent fasting enthusiasts. These virtual spaces can offer the support and information you need to feel confident in your fasting journey.

Offline, local health or wellness groups often include members who practice intermittent fasting. Many cities have meetup groups for those interested in health and wellness, which can be found through websites like Meetup.com. Joining these groups can provide a sense of community and also the opportunity to make new friends who share your interests. Additionally, consider starting your own fasting circle among friends or colleagues. This can not only enhance your social relationships but also provide a built-in support system where you can share tips, meals, and encouragement.

Engaging family and friends in your fasting journey can also enhance your experience. They may not join you in fasting, but their understanding and support can make a significant difference. Educate them about why you've chosen this path: the health benefits you hope to achieve and how it works. This understanding can help them provide the emotional support you need and respect your eating schedule, particularly during shared meals. If they're curious, invite them to join you for a fasting challenge.

This can turn a personal health endeavour into a fun, communal experience, enhancing your relationship through shared goals.

For personalised guidance, consider professional support from dietitians, health coaches, or therapists who are knowledgeable about intermittent fasting. These professionals can provide tailored advice based on your health needs, preferences, and lifestyle. They can help you fine-tune your fasting plan, suggest nutritional adjustments, and support you through emotional or psychological challenges that may arise. Their expertise can be particularly valuable when you're starting out or when you encounter hurdles in your fasting journey.

In building your support network, remember that every interaction and relationship contributes to a web of support that can hold you steady on your path. This network not only enhances your success in intermittent fasting but also enriches your life, providing deeper connections and a shared journey toward better health. As you continue to weave these connections, you'll find that the strength of your network reflects back on you, offering support, motivation, and shared joy in your achievements.

In summary, Chapter 5 has explored the multifaceted ways in which intermittent fasting can be integrated into your life, enhancing not only your physical health but your mental and emotional well-being. From the psychological boosts of improved mental clarity and mood stability to the physical benefits of mindful eating and tailored exercise, each aspect contributes to a comprehensive approach to wellness. We've seen how hydration plays a critical role in supporting your fasting and overall health, and how effective stress management can enhance your fasting success. Lastly, the value of a supportive community - whether found online, in local groups, or among friends and family - reinforces that the journey of health is one best shared. As we turn the page to the next chapter, we'll delve into how intermittent fasting influences long-term health outcomes, preparing you to not only continue this path but to thrive on it. Simply taking the time to give a review of this book helps others to understand the benefits of fasting and can join you on this journey.

Chapter 6

Beyond Weight Loss: The Health Benefits of Intermittent Fasting

As the golden hues of sunrise promise a new day, so too does your journey with intermittent fasting promise a renewal of health, especially concerning your heart's vitality. Often, the spotlight on intermittent fasting highlights its prowess in weight management, yet its influence extends profoundly into the realm of cardiovascular health - a prime concern for many women over 50. This chapter aims to peel back the layers of how this simple, yet powerful, dietary approach goes beyond mere weight loss to fortify the very engine of your body: your heart.

Intermittent Fasting & Cardiovascular Health

The heart, a tireless dynamo upon which every beat of life depends, demands our attention and care, particularly as we step into the later chapters of our lives. Intermittent fasting emerges not just as a dietary choice but as a beacon of hope for enhancing heart health. By incorporating fasting into your routine, you are stepping into a practice that can significantly diminish the risk factors associated with cardiovascular disease, the leading cause of death among women globally.

Reducing Heart Disease Risk

The mechanics of how intermittent fasting influences heart health are as intricate as they are beneficial. One of the most direct impacts is the reduction of high blood pressure, a notorious risk factor for heart disease. Regular fasting helps to regulate blood pressure by improving the elasticity of blood vessels and reducing inflammation, two factors that are often exacerbated by continuous eating patterns. Furthermore, intermittent fasting optimises lipid profiles - notably by decreasing the levels of triglycerides and low-density lipoprotein (LDL) cholesterol, known colloquially as 'bad cholesterol'. These lipids are pivotal in the buildup of plaques in arteries, which can lead to atherosclerosis, a critical pathway to heart disease. By fasting, you encourage your body to burn these lipids for energy, clearing them from your system and reducing their detrimental impact on your cardiovascular health.

Enhancing Blood Vessel Health

The health of your blood vessels is central to overall cardiovascular health. Intermittent fasting positively affects endothelial function, which is the ability of your blood vessels to contract and expand as needed. This flexibility of the vessels is crucial for maintaining proper blood flow and pressure. During fasting, there is a significant reduction in oxidative stress and inflammation - two major enemies of endothelial function. This not only helps in maintaining the elasticity of the blood vessels but also prevents the various heart diseases that can arise from compromised vascular health.

Regulating Cholesterol Levels

Managing cholesterol levels is a significant concern for many, especially post-menopausal women who may experience natural shifts in body fat distribution and metabolism, leading to elevated cholesterol levels. Intermittent fasting acts as a modulator of cholesterol by enhancing the liver's ability to process fats. It increases the levels of high-density lipoprotein (HDL), commonly known as 'good cholesterol,' which plays a role in transporting fats away from the arteries to the liver for processing. Simultaneously, it reduces the levels of LDL cholesterol, thereby striking a balance that is conducive to heart health.

Practical Heart-Healthy Fasting Tips

To harness the full potential of intermittent fasting for cardiovascular health, consider timing your exercise to coincide with your fasting state. Engaging in cardio exercises, such as brisk walking or cycling, before your first meal can enhance fat utilisation and boost circulation, maximising the heart-health benefits of your fasting regimen. Additionally, focus on hydration and electrolyte balance during fasting periods to maintain blood volume and pressure, ensuring your heart is not under undue stress due to dehydration.

Incorporating these strategies into your intermittent fasting routine can transform a simple dietary adjustment into a powerful tool for heart health. As you continue to explore the multifaceted benefits of intermittent fasting, remember that each step you take is not just about prolonging life but enhancing the quality of every heartbeat.

Cognitive Function & Brain Health

As you continue to explore the myriad of benefits offered by intermittent fasting, one particularly exciting aspect is its profound impact on cognitive function and brain health. The brain, a hub of complex activity, requires optimal conditions for its maintenance and growth. Intermittent fasting aids this by promoting the production of neurotrophic factors - proteins that are crucial for neuron growth and the survival of existing neurons. These proteins, including Brain-Derived Neurotrophic Factor (BDNF), are vital for enhancing cognitive abilities and protecting the brain against degeneration. BDNF, in particular, plays a pivotal role in memory, learning, and higher thinking processes, and its levels are significantly increased in response to the metabolic changes induced by fasting. This increase not only helps in maintaining the health of nerve cells but also stimulates the growth of new neurons and the formation of synapses, the junctions through which neurons communicate.

The potential of intermittent fasting to delay the onset and progression of neurodegenerative diseases is grounded in its capacity to improve the body's mechanisms for removing waste and toxins from cells, a process known as autophagy. Enhanced autophagy is beneficial for brain cells, as it helps clear out damaged and dysfunctional components, such as misfolded proteins associated with diseases like Alzheimer's and Parkinson's. By promoting better waste clearance, intermittent fasting helps maintain the cleanliness and efficiency of brain cells, potentially delaying or reducing the severity of neurodegenerative diseases. This protective effect is further supported by the reduction in inflammation and oxidative stress that fasting encourages, both of which are known contributors to cognitive decline and brain ageing.

In addition to protecting the brain from degenerative diseases, intermittent fasting has shown promising results in enhancing various aspects of cognitive function, including memory, focus, and the speed of information processing. These improvements are often attributed to the metabolic switch from glucose-based to ketone-based energy that occurs during fasting periods. Ketones, being more efficient and cleaner energy sources for the brain than glucose, help improve mental clarity and cognitive efficiency. They provide a steady source of energy that avoids the peaks and troughs associated with fluctuating blood sugar levels, leading to enhanced concentration and mental performance.

To further support brain health during your eating windows, incorporating specific nutrients and foods is essential.

Omega-3 fatty acids, particularly those found in fish like salmon and sardines, are renowned for their anti-inflammatory properties and their role in building and maintaining the integrity of the brain cell membranes. Anti-oxidants, found abundantly in berries, leafy greens, and nuts, protect the brain from oxidative stress and inflammation, both of which can contribute to cognitive decline. The meat from ruminants such as beef and lamb, bone broth that heals the intestinal walls, known as leaky gut, with multicoloured vegetables all contribute to a sense of wellbeing. These nutrients, when included as part of a balanced diet in your eating windows, complement the brain-boosting benefits of intermittent fasting, ensuring that your brain receives all the necessary tools to function optimally.

By understanding and leveraging the cognitive and neuroprotective benefits of intermittent fasting, you empower yourself not only to enhance your mental acuity but also to protect your brain health as you age. This approach goes beyond traditional dietary adjustments, offering a holistic strategy that supports both the body and the mind, ensuring that your later years are not only longer but are spent with a healthier, more vibrant brain.

Intermittent Fasting's Role in Cancer Prevention

As we navigate the complexities of ageing and health, one formidable aspect that often surfaces with increasing concern is the risk of cancer. Intermittent fasting has emerged not only as a method for managing weight and enhancing metabolic health but also as a potential ally in cancer prevention and treatment. Understanding how this dietary approach influences cancer risk factors and cell cycles can provide invaluable insights, empowering you with strategies to potentially lower your cancer risk and support your body during treatment, should the need arise. Trials are underway to determine the benefits of fasting during chemotherapy and so far we have found that it greatly reduces side effects.

Reducing Cancer Risk Factors

At the core of intermittent fasting's benefits in cancer prevention is its impact on insulin resistance, inflammation, and obesity - three significant cancer risk factors. Elevated insulin levels and insulin resistance have been linked to several types of cancer, including breast and endometrial cancer, which are particularly relevant for women over 50.

Intermittent fasting improves insulin sensitivity, thereby reducing insulin levels and the associated growth signals that can accelerate cancer cell growth. Moreover, the anti-inflammatory effects of fasting are profound, as chronic inflammation is a known contributor to the cancer development process. By reducing inflammation, intermittent fasting helps mitigate one of the critical environments that foster cancer cell proliferation. Additionally, the weight loss typically associated with intermittent fasting can decrease the body fat that secretes oestrogen and inflammatory markers, further reducing cancer risk.

Impact on Cell Cycles

The influence of intermittent fasting extends to the cellular level, impacting cell cycles in ways that can inhibit cancer progression. Research has shown that fasting can induce changes in the growth hormone pathways that cancer cells exploit to grow. By altering these pathways, intermittent fasting can slow cancer cell growth and even trigger programmed cell death, known as apoptosis, in cancerous cells. This cellular clean-up process is crucial as it helps the body rid itself of potentially harmful cells. Another aspect of fasting's impact on cell cycles is its ability to enhance DNA repair mechanisms and improve the cells' ability to cope with DNA damage, which is often a precursor to cancer. These protective effects not only reduce the likelihood of cancer development but also suppress the advancement of existing cancer cells.

Enhancing the Effectiveness of Chemotherapy

For those undergoing chemotherapy, intermittent fasting might offer additional benefits by enhancing the treatment's effectiveness. Studies have suggested that fasting can make cancer cells more susceptible to chemotherapy while simultaneously protecting normal, healthy cells from the toxic effects of cancer treatments. This differential protection, known as differential stress resistance, can result in fewer side effects and improved cancer cell targeting during chemotherapy. The theory is that fasting stresses cancer cells, which are less adaptable than normal cells, making them more vulnerable to treatments that target fast-growing cells. At the same time, fasting induces a protective state in normal cells, which helps them resist the stress of chemotherapy drugs, potentially leading to a better patient experience and outcomes.

Precautions & Guidance

While the benefits of intermittent fasting in the context of cancer prevention and treatment are promising, it is crucial to approach this practice with caution and informed guidance. If you have a history of cancer or are at high risk, it is imperative to consult with your healthcare provider rather than going it alone. More and more doctors and naturopaths like myself are using fasting as a preventative, help spread the word by looking at the results of research and trials and making sure that your health care provider is aware of this information. They can provide personalised advice that considers your overall health, medical history, and specific cancer risk factors. Additionally, monitoring your body's response to fasting is essential, as individual reactions can vary.

Embracing intermittent fasting as part of your cancer prevention strategy or as a complementary approach during cancer treatment provides a proactive stance against one of the most challenging diseases. By understanding and leveraging the multifaceted benefits of intermittent fasting, you are not only taking a step towards reducing cancer risk but also enhancing your body's resilience and capacity to thrive in the face of adversity. As you continue to explore the potential of intermittent fasting, remember that each choice you make is a part of nurturing a healthier, more empowered self.

Diabetes Management & Prevention Strategies

In the landscape of health concerns that touch many of us as we navigate our golden years, diabetes stands out due to its wide-reaching implications on overall well-being. Particularly for women over 50, managing or even preventing type 2 diabetes becomes crucial as the body undergoes metabolic and hormonal changes. Intermittent fasting, a practice deeply woven with the rhythms of our ancestral heritage, emerges here as a modern tool with profound benefits for insulin regulation and blood sugar management.

Improving Insulin Sensitivity

The crux of managing and preventing diabetes revolves significantly around insulin sensitivity. This term refers to how effectively your body's cells respond to insulin, the hormone responsible for shuttling glucose from your bloodstream into your cells where it's used for energy. With age, particularly after menopause, many women experience a decline in insulin sensitivity, a condition often exacerbated by increased adipose tissue and decreased muscle mass. Intermittent fasting steps into this scenario as a potent modulator of insulin sensitivity. By alternating between periods of eating and fasting, your body learns to utilise insulin more efficiently. During fasting periods, insulin levels drop significantly, prompting your cells to increase their sensitivity to insulin. This adaptation can have a lasting impact, improving your body's ability to manage glucose levels and reducing the risk of type 2 diabetes. The shift to burning fat for fuel during fasting periods also plays a pivotal role, as it decreases fat stores, linked directly to improved insulin sensitivity.

Regulating Blood Sugar Levels

Stabilising blood sugar levels is another arena where intermittent fasting exhibits its strengths. Fluctuations in blood sugar levels can create a rollercoaster of energy highs and lows, exacerbating not only diabetes symptoms but also influencing hunger and satiety. Intermittent fasting helps smooth out these fluctuations by enhancing hormonal balance and fostering a metabolic environment where the body becomes more adept at using fat for energy, a process that produces fewer rapid spikes in blood sugar compared to carbohydrate metabolism. For women dealing with the erratic hormonal shifts that accompany menopause, this stabilisation can mean not just better management of diabetes but also an improvement in overall energy levels and mood.

Fasting Protocols for Diabetics

While the benefits of intermittent fasting for diabetes management are compelling, it's crucial that such a regimen is approached with care, especially if you are already diagnosed with diabetes. Tailored advice on safely engaging in intermittent fasting often includes close monitoring by healthcare providers. If you're using IF to reverse diabetes it is good to find an expert in fasting and if you can't find one near you there is help from experts over zoom. Together, you might develop a monitored approach where you gradually increase fasting intervals, carefully observing how your blood sugar responds. Continuous glucose monitoring devices can be invaluable in this regard, providing real-time feedback and helping adjust your fasting schedule to optimise blood sugar control.

Lifestyle Integration

Finally, integrating intermittent fasting with other lifestyle strategies can amplify its benefits and support robust diabetes management. Regular physical activity, for example, not only boosts insulin sensitivity further but also helps regulate blood sugar levels more directly by increasing glucose uptake by muscles during and after exercise. Stress reduction techniques such as yoga, meditation, or even simple breathing exercises can also play a supportive role. Stress hormones such as cortisol can interfere with insulin sensitivity and glucose control. By incorporating practices that mitigate stress, you enhance your body's ability to manage diabetes effectively. Combining these strategies with intermittent fasting creates a comprehensive approach to diabetes care that aligns with your body's natural rhythms and healing capabilities, promoting not just longevity but a higher quality of life.

As you navigate these strategies, remember that the goal is to create a sustainable, enjoyable lifestyle that not only addresses diabetes management or prevention but also enhances your overall well-being. With each meal, each fast, and each step or breath you take, you are nurturing a body that has supported you through decades of life's challenges and joys. Let the wisdom of intermittent fasting guide you to a healthier, more vibrant future where diabetes does not dictate your choices but rather informs how you live well.

Improving Digestive Health Through Fasting

In the rhythm of our lives, where each meal often seamlessly leads into another, there's seldom a pause that allows our digestive system to rest. Intermittent fasting introduces such a pause, a respite that can bring profound benefits to digestive health, especially for women over 50 who might start experiencing increased digestive issues as their bodies continue to change. By strategically timing your eating and fasting periods, you give your digestive tract time to rest and repair, akin to how sleep rejuvenates the mind and body. This break can significantly reduce symptoms of digestive disorders such as bloating, gas, and inflammation which are not just uncomfortable but can also interfere with your daily life and well-being.

The process is quite straightforward: during fasting periods, the energy that would typically be used for digestion is redirected towards repairing tissues and cells throughout the body, including those within the gastrointestinal system. This can lead to reduced inflammation in the gut, a common culprit behind bloating and gas. Moreover, intermittent fasting can increase the production of the gut hormone ghrelin, which not only regulates hunger but also enhances gastric motility and improves digestive function. Regular fasting can thus help in maintaining a healthier, more efficient digestive system which is less prone to common issues such as indigestion and constipation.

Turning to the gut microbiome, which plays a crucial role not just in digestion but also in overall health and immunity, intermittent fasting can be a boon. The composition and health of your gut microbiota can change depending on many factors, including diet, stress, and medication. Fasting has been shown to promote the growth of beneficial gut bacteria, which can enhance gut health and strengthen the immune system. The mechanism behind this lies in the changes in gut pH and the availability of substrates during fasting, which can favour the growth of beneficial microbes over harmful ones. This shift can have widespread benefits, not only improving digestion and nutrient absorption but also enhancing metabolic health and reducing inflammation throughout the body.

As you begin to integrate intermittent fasting into your life, it's not uncommon that some digestive discomfort will resolve such as acid reflux or constipation. These issues typically arise as your body adjusts to any dietary changes and hormonal changes. To manage acid reflux, consider adjusting the timing of your last meal, ensuring that you finish eating a few hours before going to bed, thus giving your body ample time to digest the food. Elevating the head of your bed slightly can also help prevent stomach acid from travelling up the oesophagus while you sleep. For constipation, increasing your intake of water during your eating periods and throughout the fast is crucial. Hydration plays a key role in digestive health, helping to soften stools and promote regular bowel movements. Additionally, incorporating foods rich in fibre such as vegetables, avocados, salads and legumes during your eating windows can help maintain bowel health and regularity.

Balanced eating during your designated eating windows plays a pivotal role in optimising digestive health. It's not just about what you eat, but how you eat. Slow, mindful eating can significantly improve how your body digests and absorbs nutrients. Chewing thoroughly and eating in a relaxed setting can enhance enzyme secretion, making digestion smoother and more efficient. Furthermore, integrating probiotic-rich foods like yoghurt, kefir, sauerkraut, and kombucha can help maintain a healthy balance of gut bacteria, enhancing gut health and overall digestion. Prebiotic foods, which serve as food for beneficial gut bacteria, are equally important. Foods rich in prebiotic fibres like garlic, onions, avocados and asparagus can help nourish the beneficial bacteria in your gut, promoting a balanced microbiome.

By adopting these strategies, you not only ease common digestive issues but also set the stage for a healthier digestive system that supports your overall health and well-being. Intermittent fasting offers a unique approach to digestive health, emphasising the importance of when you eat and giving your body the rest it needs to repair and rejuvenate. As you continue to explore this path, remember that each step you take towards balancing your eating and fasting periods is a step towards a healthier, more vibrant digestive system.

Longevity & Life Extension: What the Research Says

The quest for a long and healthy life is as old as humanity itself. Intermittent fasting, with its deep roots in human history, is now being recognized through modern science as a potent ally in this quest. The mechanisms by which intermittent fasting is believed to enhance longevity are multifaceted and profound, involving reduced oxidative stress, enhanced cellular repair processes, and significant improvements in metabolic health. These mechanisms collectively contribute to slowing down the ageing process and extending lifespan, offering you a powerful tool to not just live longer, but better.

Reduced oxidative stress is one of the primary benefits of intermittent fasting related to longevity. Oxidative stress occurs when there is an imbalance between free radicals and antioxidants in your body, leading to cell damage. Intermittent fasting helps reduce oxidative stress by enhancing the body's antioxidant defences and decreasing the production of free radicals. This reduction in oxidative stress is crucial for preventing age-related diseases and degeneration, thereby potentially extending lifespan. Moreover, intermittent fasting stimulates autophagy, a cellular cleanup process that removes damaged and dysfunctional proteins and organelles. This process is vital for cellular health and longevity, as it helps prevent the accumulation of cellular debris that can lead to senescence and the development of various diseases.

The impact of intermittent fasting on metabolic health also plays a significant role in its ability to extend life. By improving insulin sensitivity and reducing inflammation, intermittent fasting can mitigate the risk factors associated with metabolic syndrome, including obesity, hypertension, and diabetes, all of which can significantly shorten lifespan. Furthermore, intermittent fasting has been shown to enhance hormone function, including the hormones involved in growth and metabolism, which are crucial for maintaining youthfulness and vitality.

Research on fasting and longevity provides compelling evidence of its benefits. Various studies involving animal models have shown that intermittent fasting can extend lifespan significantly. For instance, research on rodents has demonstrated that intermittent fasting can increase lifespan by approximately 30%, a remarkable figure that has spurred further research into its applicability in humans. While direct evidence in humans is more challenging to ascertain due to the long lifespans and ethical considerations, observational studies and shorter-term human trials have shown promising results, such as improved biomarkers of longevity and reduced signs of ageing.

To incorporate intermittent fasting into your lifestyle effectively, a balanced approach is essential. This includes integrating nutritious foods during your eating windows to ensure your body receives all the necessary nutrients to support health and longevity. Focus on a diet rich in vegetables, good fats and animal proteins, and consider incorporating supplements as needed to address any nutritional gaps. Additionally, regular exercise should be a cornerstone of your routine, as physical activity not only complements the benefits of fasting but also directly contributes to longer life by improving heart health, strengthening bones and muscles, and enhancing mental health.

In summary, intermittent fasting holds remarkable potential for extending lifespan and enhancing the quality of life. By reducing oxidative stress, enhancing cellular repair, and improving metabolic health, this age-old practice offers modern-day benefits that align with the goals of living a longer, healthier life. As you explore the potential of intermittent fasting for longevity, remember that a balanced, informed approach is key to harnessing its full benefits. Let this knowledge guide you as you continue to explore ways to enhance your health and vitality through diet, exercise, and mindful living.

As we conclude this exploration of intermittent fasting's role in longevity and life extension, remember that the journey to a healthier, longer life is multifaceted. Intermittent fasting is a powerful tool in your arsenal, but it is most effective when combined with a holistic approach to health that includes balanced nutrition, regular physical activity, and mindful stress management. In the next chapter, we will delve into practical strategies for integrating intermittent fasting into your daily life, ensuring that you can apply these insights in a way that fits your unique lifestyle and health goals.

Chapter 7

Real Life Success Stories

Every transformation begins with a story of change, and the most compelling ones often start with doubt. This is certainly true in the world of intermittent fasting, where every successful journey shines as a beacon of possibility and hope. It's through these narratives that you can see the tangible impact of intermittent fasting, not just in numbers on a scale but in real, lived experiences. Let's explore these journeys, starting with Jane, who transformed from a sceptic to a staunch advocate for intermittent fasting.

From Sceptic to Believer: Jane's Journey

Jane's initial encounter with intermittent fasting was steeped in scepticism. Having navigated a maze of diet trends that promised much but delivered little, she approached fasting with a hefty dose of wariness. Her past dieting failures had left a residue of disappointment, and the prevalent myths around fasting - that it was just another fad only fueled her doubts. However, it was her friend's transformation that piqued her curiosity and prompted her to delve deeper, challenging her own misconceptions.

The turning point for Jane came when she attended a workshop that demystified intermittent fasting with robust scientific evidence and testimonials. The session covered various studies that highlighted the benefits of fasting not just for weight loss but for metabolic health, hormonal balance, and even mental clarity. Learning about the body's response to fasting - how it switches to fat burning and enhances cellular repair during fasting periods - Jane began to see intermittent fasting in a new light. The idea that fasting could help reset her body and potentially reverse some of the age-related decline was both intriguing and motivating.

With newfound knowledge and cautious optimism, Jane started her intermittent fasting journey with an 8-hour eating window. The early days were challenging. Hunger pangs and old habits urged her to reach for snacks outside her eating window, but armed with strategies like hydrating well, staying busy during fasting periods, and focusing on nutrient-dense foods during her eating window, she slowly adapted. Jane also started journaling her experience, a practice that not only helped her track her progress but also became a reflective tool for understanding her relationship with food.

Visual Element: Jane's Fasting Tracker

A sample page from Jane's journal shows her fasting schedule, her emotional and physical feelings noted during different phases, and her dietary intake, providing a real-world example of how tracking can aid in the fasting process.

Over months, Jane noticed significant changes. She lost weight, yes, but more importantly, she felt more energetic, her sleep quality improved, and her blood pressure readings lowered. Her success with intermittent fasting transformed her from a sceptic to a believer, a journey she was eager to share. She started by initiating conversations in her social circles, gradually becoming a local advocate in her community. She hosted informational sessions, sharing her story and the evidence behind fasting, helping to dispel myths and inspire others, especially women over fifty who thought their days of feeling vibrant and healthy were behind them.

Today, Jane's routine includes a flexible fasting schedule that she adjusts according to her body's needs and her social commitments. Her advocacy for intermittent fasting is driven by her personal experience and the deep belief in its benefits, supported by ongoing research. She continues to engage with fasting communities online and locally, spreading knowledge and supporting others in their journeys.

Jane's story is a testament to the transformative power of intermittent fasting, underscored by personal experience and scientific support. It reflects a journey of overcoming initial doubts and embracing a lifestyle change that brought not just improved health but also a renewed sense of control and empowerment. Her story, like many others, illustrates that with the right information, support, and a willingness to adapt, the benefits of intermittent fasting can indeed be a reality, especially for women navigating the complexities of health after fifty.

Reversing Diabetes with IF: Lisa's Story

When Lisa was first diagnosed with type 2 diabetes, it wasn't just a wake-up call; it was a loud siren demanding immediate attention. Her daily life had become a series of strict routines: monitoring blood sugar levels, taking multiple medications, and trying to control her weight, which seemed an uphill battle. Complications like fatigue, nerve pain, and the looming risk of cardiovascular disease made every day a challenge. With a family history of diabetes and heart disease, Lisa knew she had to find a sustainable solution that not only addressed her symptoms but also the root cause of her health issues.

Under the guidance of her endocrinologist, Lisa began exploring intermittent fasting as part of a comprehensive management plan for her diabetes. The idea was initially daunting - forgoing food for extended periods seemed counterintuitive, especially for someone who needed to keep her blood sugar levels stable. However, her doctor explained that with careful monitoring and a tailored approach, intermittent fasting could potentially help improve her insulin sensitivity and facilitate weight loss. They decided on a 16/8 fasting protocol, where Lisa would fast for 16 hours and have an 8-hour window for eating. This method was integrated with her existing medication regimen, which was adjusted to accommodate her new eating schedule. Lisa also received nutritional counselling to ensure her eating periods were filled with balanced meals, focusing on fibre-rich vegetables, lean proteins, and healthy fats, which would help manage her blood sugar levels more effectively.

The changes didn't happen overnight, but Lisa was committed. She started noticing that her fasting periods were not as daunting as she had anticipated. With the support of her healthcare team, she learned to recognize true hunger cues and differentiate them from habitual eating patterns. This awareness, combined with her scheduled eating times, helped Lisa gain control over her cravings and snacking habits. Over the months, this new way of eating seemed to recalibrate her body's hunger signals and energy usage. One of the most significant improvements was in her blood sugar levels. They began to stabilise within just a few weeks of starting her fasting regimen, and her need for insulin injections decreased substantially. Her endocrinologist was impressed by the improvement in her HbA1c levels, a key indicator of long-term blood glucose control, which had dropped to within near-normal ranges.

Lisa's journey with intermittent fasting transformed her from a passive observer of her health condition to an active participant in her wellness. Her energy levels improved, allowing her to enjoy activities she had avoided before due to fatigue and joint pain. She also experienced noticeable weight loss, which further improved her mobility and reduced her risk of cardiovascular complications. The physical changes were evident, but for Lisa, the true success lay in the empowerment she felt. Managing her diabetes was no longer about just following doctor's orders; it was about actively shaping her health and future.

Eager to share her success and the knowledge she had gained, Lisa turned to community involvement and online platforms. She started speaking at local health seminars, sharing her story and the positive impact intermittent fasting had on her diabetes management. Online, she became an active member of several diabetes management forums, offering advice and support to others struggling with similar issues. Her firsthand experience, backed by the noticeable improvements in her health, made her a credible and inspirational figure in these communities.

Lisa's story is a powerful example of how lifestyle changes, specifically intermittent fasting, can be effectively integrated into diabetes management under proper medical supervision. Her experience highlights the importance of personalised care and the potential for individuals to reclaim control over their health, even in the face of chronic conditions like diabetes. As more people like Lisa share their successes, intermittent fasting is gaining recognition not just for weight management but as a viable part of diabetes care, challenging long-held conventions and offering hope for a healthier life.

A New Lease on Life: Mary's Weight Loss Adventure

Mary's struggle with obesity was a long-standing battle, one that intensified as she transitioned through menopause. With hormonal changes altering her metabolism and energy levels, what used to be minor weight fluctuations turned into a steady weight gain. This wasn't just a matter of numbers on a scale; it was a profound issue that affected her mobility, her health, and her self-esteem. Simple tasks became daunting. Climbing stairs or walking her dog left her breathless, and the reflection in the mirror started to affect her more deeply, chipping away at her confidence. Each failed diet and health regimen only deepened her sense of despair, reinforcing the fear that this weight issue might be an unchangeable aspect of her ageing process.

However, Mary's introduction to intermittent fasting came at a time when she was nearly ready to give up. It was a chance conversation at a community health fair that sparked her interest. Unlike the restrictive diets she had tried before, intermittent fasting offered a different approach - one that focused on when to eat rather than obsessing over every calorie. The simplicity of the method appealed to her, and the stories of people who had found success with it ignited a flicker of hope. She decided to give it a try, adopting a 16/8 fasting protocol where she would eat all her meals within an eight-hour window and fast for the remaining sixteen. This structure, surprisingly, fit quite well into her daily routine, allowing her to skip breakfast, which she often found herself forcing down in the belief that it was the 'most important meal of the day' (a concept from a Kellogg's ad).

The first few weeks were challenging, as her body adjusted to the new eating pattern. Feelings of hunger and cravings were intense as her usual meal times approached, but Mary found support through an online community of intermittent fasters. The group, consisting of individuals from various age groups and walks of life, shared their experiences and tips, which were invaluable in helping Mary navigate her initial struggles. They discussed everything from how to handle social meals to what nutrient-dense foods were best during eating windows to maximise satiety and nutrition. This support system was crucial in keeping Mary motivated and reminding her that the discomfort was temporary and part of the adjustment phase.

As weeks turned into months, Mary began to notice significant changes. The scale started to reflect her efforts, but more importantly, her energy levels increased. She found herself enjoying walks in the park, noticing less joint pain and an improved mood. These changes were not just physical; they were emotional and psychological. With each pound lost, she gained confidence, not just in her appearance but in her ability to control her health destiny. This empowerment was a new feeling, one that she cherished deeply.

Mary's transformation was profound. Over a year into her intermittent fasting lifestyle, she had not only lost significant weight but had maintained her new weight with ease, something she had never managed to do with previous diets. Her success with intermittent fasting rekindled her love for outdoor activities, leading her to take up hiking - a hobby she had abandoned in her younger years due to her weight. The joy of reaching a summit, which she once thought was lost to her, became a regular celebration of her new capabilities and her body's resilience.

Moreover, Mary's journey inspired her to help others. She began speaking at local health seminars, sharing her story from the perspective of someone who had lived through the struggle of obesity and emerged healthier and happier. Her talks were filled not just with practical advice about intermittent fasting but with encouragement and empathy for those who felt trapped by their weight issues. Mary's story, marked by genuine understanding and support, made her an effective advocate for healthy living and an inspiration to many who thought their age or past failures defined their health futures.

Mary's new lease on life, powered by her success with intermittent fasting, turned her golden years into some of the most vibrant and fulfilling years of her life. Her story is a testament to the power of resilience, the importance of support, and the transformative potential of rethinking how and when we eat. For Mary, and for many like her, intermittent fasting was not just a method to lose weight - it was a gateway to a renewed sense of self and a more joyful, healthful approach to life.

Balancing Hormones Naturally: Susan's Tale

Susan's midlife years brought more than just a wealth of experience and wisdom; they also ushered in a series of hormonal imbalances that disrupted her life in ways she hadn't anticipated. Hot flashes became an unwelcome intrusion, appearing at the most inconvenient times, while mood swings turned her once-stable temperament into something more unpredictable. Nights were the worst, as insomnia frequently kept her from the restorative sleep she desperately needed. Like many women her age, Susan found herself wrestling with the physical and emotional rollercoaster of menopause, feeling at the mercy of her fluctuating hormones.

In her search for relief, Susan stumbled upon intermittent fasting almost by accident, during a health and wellness conference she attended more or less out of curiosity. Intrigued by preliminary research suggesting that intermittent fasting could help regulate hormones naturally, she dove deeper. She learned that the fasting process could potentially stabilise insulin levels, reduce inflammation, and even influence hormone function, all of which could play a crucial role in alleviating her menopausal symptoms. The science made sense to her; by giving her body a break from digesting food, she could allow it to focus more on other essential functions, including hormone regulation.

Armed with this knowledge, Susan approached her healthcare provider to discuss the possibility of integrating intermittent fasting into her lifestyle. With guidance, she decided on a 16/8 fasting protocol, which involved fasting for 16 hours each day and eating her meals within an eight-hour window. This schedule meant she could have dinner early in the evening and then skip breakfast, a meal she never felt much desire for anyway, making the transition smoother than she had anticipated. Her doctor also advised her to keep a detailed log of her symptoms and dietary intake, which helped them both monitor her progress and adjust her plan as needed.

The effects of this new eating pattern on her hormonal symptoms were gradual but undeniable. Within a few months, Susan noticed a significant reduction in the frequency and intensity of her hot flashes and emotional stability seemed to fortify. Even her sleep improved, which she hadn't dared hope for when she started. These changes were not just subjective feelings; they were also reflected in her medical check-ups. Her blood tests showed improved insulin sensitivity and a better inflammatory profile, indicators that her body was responding positively to her new fasting regimen.

Encouraged by these results, Susan began to embrace other lifestyle changes to enhance her health further. She increased her physical activity, adding yoga and light strength training to her routine, which not only helped her manage stress but also improved her muscle tone and joint health, both of which are crucial for ageing women. Nutrition-wise, she shifted towards a more plant-based diet, rich in vegetables, fruits, whole grains, and healthy fats, which complemented her fasting schedule and supported her overall well-being. These dietary choices were aimed not just at weight management but at enriching her body with the nutrients needed to support hormonal balance and cognitive function.

Susan's holistic approach to managing her health in midlife through intermittent fasting and supportive lifestyle adjustments became a testament to the power of proactive well-being. Her experience, marked by significant improvements in her symptoms and overall health, turned her into a vocal proponent of intermittent fasting, particularly for women grappling with hormonal imbalances. She began sharing her story, hoping to inspire other women to explore this potential path to hormonal harmony and improved quality of life. Her talks at local community centres and posts on health-focused online forums not only spread the word but also offered hope and guidance to many who thought their struggles were an inevitable part of ageing. Susan's journey illustrates the transformative impact of combining intermittent fasting with a mindful approach to lifestyle changes, offering a blueprint for managing health naturally and effectively.

Finding Community & Support: Karen's Experience

Karen's venture into the realm of health and wellness often felt like navigating a solitary path. Despite her dedication and efforts, the initial phase of her health journey was marked by profound isolation. This feeling of being alone wasn't just about lacking companionship; it was about grappling with the challenges of improving her health without support, understanding, or shared experiences. Her attempts at dieting and lifestyle changes prior to discovering intermittent fasting were punctuated by moments of struggle and frustration, which seemed magnified by the absence of someone who could relate or guide her. This solitude in her quest for health made each setback feel more personal and each failure more discouraging.

However, Karen's discovery of intermittent fasting was a pivotal moment that extended beyond learning about a new eating pattern. As she delved into this new approach, she found herself stepping into a vibrant community of like-minded individuals, both online and within her local area. Her first encounter with this supportive network came through a local health workshop focused on intermittent fasting, where she met others who were either curious about or seasoned in various fasting methods. The sense of community was palpable, and for Karen, this was a revelation. She realised that her journey didn't have to be a lonely one; there were others who shared similar struggles and aspirations.

Engaging with these intermittent fasting groups opened a new world for Karen. Online forums and local meet-up groups became her regular sources of inspiration and knowledge.

These platforms allowed her to connect with people from all walks of life, each bringing their own unique perspectives and experiences with fasting. The stories shared within these groups were not just motivational; they were educational. Karen learned practical tips for managing fasting windows, the best nutrient-dense foods to focus on during eating periods, and how to handle the social aspects of dietary changes. Perhaps more importantly, these communities provided a space for emotional support. Whenever Karen felt overwhelmed or on the verge of giving up, there was always someone to offer encouragement or advice. This network of support played a crucial role in helping her maintain her commitment to intermittent fasting, transforming her initial attempts into a sustained practice.

The impact of this community support was profound, not just in how Karen managed her fasting schedule, but in how she viewed her health journey. It was no longer about just personal gain; it was about shared growth and collective well-being. This realisation inspired Karen to give back to the community that had given her so much. She started by organising local meetups for her intermittent fasting group, creating opportunities for members to connect in person, share meals, and discuss their experiences and challenges. These gatherings quickly became a cherished part of her routine, enriching her experience and strengthening the bonds within the community.

Furthermore, Karen took her engagement a step further by starting a blog dedicated to her intermittent fasting journey. The blog began as a personal project to document her progress and share insights, but it quickly grew into a valuable resource for others exploring intermittent fasting. Through her posts, Karen shared everything from recipe ideas and fasting tips to reflections on the emotional aspects of health transformation. Her honest and relatable writing style resonated with many, turning her blog into a platform for connection and discussion. Readers from around the globe reached out to share their stories and seek advice, expanding Karen's impact far beyond her local community.

Karen's experience highlights the transformative power of community in the realm of health and wellness. What started as an individual pursuit of better health evolved into a collaborative journey marked by shared experiences, collective learning, and mutual support. For Karen, and many like her, finding community within the intermittent fasting world was not just about adhering to an eating schedule; it was about connecting with others, sharing in the struggles and triumphs, and ultimately, contributing to a larger dialogue about health and well-being. Through her active participation and contribution, Karen not only enhanced her own life but also enriched the lives of others, embodying the true spirit of community and support in the journey toward better health.

The Family That Fasts Together: A Multi-Generational Story

In the tapestry of health and wellness narratives, the story of a family embracing intermittent fasting together weaves a particularly vibrant thread. This family, consisting of grandparents, their children, and teenage grandchildren, found themselves at a crossroads faced with various health issues ranging from mild obesity to high cholesterol and elevated blood sugar levels. Concerned about the legacy of health they were passing down and inspired by emerging research on the benefits of intermittent fasting, they collectively decided to test whether this lifestyle could be the key to improving their overall health.

Each family member approached intermittent fasting with their unique needs and lifestyle in mind, which meant customising their fasting schedules to fit individual routines and health goals. The grandparents, both retired, found that a 14/10 fasting schedule worked best, allowing them a leisurely breakfast and early dinner, which also helped them manage their type 2 diabetes more effectively. Their son, juggling a hectic job and parenting, opted for the 16/8 method, skipping breakfast so he could enjoy dinners with his teenage children. The grandchildren, active in sports and school activities, adopted a lighter version of fasting, restricting their eating to a 12-hour window to better accommodate their high energy demands and school schedules.

As the weeks turned into months, the family began to notice significant health improvements. The grandparents were thrilled with their improved glycemic control and reduced reliance on diabetes medication. The father noticed a marked improvement in his energy levels and a welcome reduction in his cholesterol levels, while the teenagers reported better concentration in school and enhanced performance in sports. However, these benefits were not without their challenges. Adapting to a new eating schedule required significant adjustment, particularly on holidays and family gatherings where food was a central feature. Moreover, finding meals that catered to the varied tastes and nutritional needs of three generations occasionally stirred up tensions.

Yet, these challenges were small compared to the profound bonding experience that came with sharing a commitment to healthier living. Meal planning became a collaborative effort that not only improved their diets but also brought them closer together, turning mealtime into a shared project rooted in mutual support and care. This togetherness was fortified by regular family meetings to discuss progress, swap recipes, and strategize around upcoming events, ensuring everyone stayed on track and felt supported.

The impact of their collective effort rippled beyond their immediate family. Friends, neighbours, and extended relatives took note of the visible changes in their health and vitality, sparking conversations about nutrition and preventive health. The family became informal ambassadors of intermittent fasting, sharing their success and the practical insights they had gained. Their story became a powerful testament to the potential of shared dietary strategies to not only enhance individual health but also strengthen family bonds and community connections.

This family's journey with intermittent fasting highlights the transformative potential of a unified approach to health and wellness. Their experience underscores the importance of adaptability, support, and collective commitment in navigating the challenges and reaping the substantial benefits of intermittent fasting. It serves as an inspiring example for other families considering this lifestyle change, demonstrating that with mutual support and tailored approaches, it is possible to significantly enhance not just personal health but also familial and community well-being.

As we wrap up this chapter, we reflect on the diverse stories shared, each underscoring a unique aspect of intermittent fasting's impact. From reversing chronic conditions and managing weight to restoring hormonal balance and fostering community support, these narratives illustrate the broad spectrum of benefits that intermittent fasting offers. They not only provide practical insights and inspiration but also highlight the profound personal transformations that can occur when individuals take proactive steps toward enhancing their health. As we turn the page to the next chapter, we carry forward the understanding that intermittent fasting is life changing.

Chapter 8

Sustaining & Advancing Your Intermittent Fasting Lifestyle

As you gracefully move through the different phases of life, your body undergoes numerous transformations, each requiring you to adapt and sometimes reinvent your approach to health and wellness. Intermittent fasting, which may have served you well during one season, might need adjustments as new challenges and physical changes emerge. This chapter is dedicated to ensuring that your fasting regimen evolves with you, continuing to offer health benefits and fitting seamlessly into your lifestyle as you age.

Innovating Your Fasting Regime as You Age

Adapting to Physical Changes

As you continue on your path of intermittent fasting, it's essential to recognize and adapt to the changes your body naturally experiences. You may notice a gradual decline in metabolism and a shift in energy levels as you age. These changes are not just inevitable parts of ageing but are also signals that your fasting regimen needs reassessment and adjustment. For instance, the fasting intervals that once felt invigorating might now feel overly taxing. This is a cue to consider shorter fasts or altering your fasting schedule to earlier in the day when your energy levels are higher.

Adapting your fasting routine to these changes is not about easing off but rather fine-tuning the process to align with your body's current needs. For example, if you find your energy waning during longer fasts, incorporating nutrient-dense foods like avocados and nuts during your eating windows can help sustain your energy levels throughout the day. Also, consider the timing of your last meal of the day to ensure it provides adequate nutrition to support overnight metabolic processes, which can help maintain energy levels and prevent morning fatigue.

Incorporating Preventative Measures

Preventative health measures become increasingly important as you age. Regular health screenings can help catch and address potential health issues early, but your diet, particularly in how you structure your intermittent fasting, plays a crucial role as well. Dietary adjustments to accommodate specific needs such as increased calcium for bone density or higher fibre intake for digestive health are essential.

Moreover, consider the quality of your diet during eating windows. It's not just about what you avoid eating but also about what you actively include. Foods rich in antioxidants, for example, can help combat inflammation, a common issue as the body ages. Integrating such preventative dietary strategies can significantly impact your overall well-being, making your intermittent fasting routine a powerful ally in maintaining your health.

Exploring Longer Fasting Periods

For those who have been practising intermittent fasting successfully and are curious about deepening their practice, exploring longer fasting periods can be beneficial. Extended fasts, such as 24-hour fasts, once or twice a week, have been shown to enhance the benefits of cellular repair and autophagy - your body's way of cleaning out damaged cells to regenerate newer, healthier cells. However, it's crucial to approach this practice with caution, especially as your body's resilience might change with age.

Start slowly, perhaps with a trial fast extending a few hours beyond your usual routine, and observe how your body responds. It's important to stay hydrated and to break your fast gently, prioritising easily digestible foods that nourish and replenish your body. If you find these extended fasts beneficial, they can be a valuable addition to your intermittent fasting regimen, potentially offering enhanced anti-aging benefits and improved metabolic health.

Continuous Learning

The landscape of nutritional science and health research is continually evolving, with new studies frequently shedding light on better practices and deeper insights into how our bodies respond to diets like intermittent fasting. Staying informed about the latest research not only helps you optimise your fasting regimen but also ensures that you are aware of any new developments that might impact your health strategy.

Subscribe to health newsletters, listen to podcasts, or even join online courses on nutrition and wellness. These resources can offer valuable information that can inspire adjustments and innovations in your fasting routine, keeping it aligned with the latest scientific understanding and best practices. Engaging with a community of like-minded individuals who are also exploring intermittent fasting can provide support and insight, making your journey into continuous learning both a personal and shared experience.

As you adapt your intermittent fasting practice to meet the evolving needs of your body and lifestyle, remember that flexibility and attentiveness to your body's signals are key. By embracing change and seeking out new knowledge, you ensure that your approach to health and wellness not only meets your current needs but also supports your vitality and well-being for years to come.

Mindset Shifts for Lifelong Fasting

Cultivating an Adaptive Mindset

Embracing intermittent fasting as a lifelong approach to health and wellness requires more than just a physical adjustment - it demands a mental shift towards flexibility and adaptability. As you age, your body and lifestyle will inevitably change, and your ability to adapt your fasting regimen to these changes is crucial for maintaining its effectiveness and ensuring it continues to bring you joy and health benefits. Think of this adaptability as a form of mental agility, a skill that allows you to navigate life's inevitable ups and downs with grace and resilience.

Developing an adaptive mindset involves seeing changes and challenges not as obstacles but as opportunities for growth and learning. For instance, if you find that your energy levels are not what they used to be, instead of viewing this as a setback, consider it a chance to explore new fasting schedules or dietary adjustments that could help boost your vitality. This might mean shifting your eating window or incorporating more nutrient-dense foods into your diet. By staying curious and open to experimenting with these adjustments, you transform your fasting practice into a dynamic tool that evolves with you, continually aligned with your body's current needs.

This mindset also extends to how you perceive intermittent fasting within the broader context of your life. It's not just a diet but a lifestyle choice that influences many aspects of your well-being - from your physical health to your mental clarity and emotional balance. Approaching fasting with a mindset that welcomes change ensures that you remain proactive about your health, ready to tweak and transform your approach as your life changes, ensuring that fasting remains a rewarding part of your life, no matter your age.

Long-term Goal Setting

Setting long-term goals is a powerful way to sustain your commitment to intermittent fasting. These goals should resonate with your deeper motivations for choosing this lifestyle - whether it's maintaining agility and strength as you age, managing a health condition, or simply wanting to live a vibrant, active life. Long-term goals provide a roadmap, guiding your choices and keeping you motivated, especially when the day-to-day challenges of fasting might feel daunting.

When setting these goals, be specific and realistic. Instead of a vague goal like 'stay healthy', pinpoint what health looks like for you. Does it mean being able to play with your grandchildren without feeling fatigued, or does it involve managing your blood sugar levels to keep diabetes at bay? Perhaps it's about maintaining mental sharpness and memory. Once these goals are clear, break them down into actionable steps. For instance, if your goal is to improve cardiovascular health, your action steps might include scheduling regular check-ups, monitoring your heart rate during exercise, and adjusting your fasting schedule to include more heart-healthy foods during your eating windows.

Keep these goals visible - write them down in a journal, create a vision board, or place reminders in your home. Seeing these reminders daily can help keep your focus aligned with your objectives, encouraging a sustained commitment to your intermittent fasting lifestyle, even when obstacles arise.

Emotional Resilience

Building emotional resilience is key to managing the ups and downs of a fasting lifestyle over the long term. Emotional resilience helps you recover from setbacks and maintain a positive outlook, even when your fasting journey becomes challenging. This resilience can be strengthened through practices like mindfulness meditation, which teaches you to stay present and calm, reducing the stress that can come with dietary changes.

Another strategy is to regularly engage in activities that boost your mood and overall mental health. Whether it's walking in nature, practising yoga, or spending time with loved ones, these activities can provide emotional uplifts that bolster your resilience. Additionally, maintaining a gratitude journal where you record not only your fasting successes but also other positive aspects of your life can shift your focus from challenges to achievements, reinforcing a positive mindset.

Celebrating Milestones

Recognizing and celebrating milestones in your intermittent fasting journey is crucial for motivation. These celebrations can be as simple as acknowledging a month of sticking with your fasting schedule or as significant as reaching a health goal like lowering your cholesterol levels. Celebrating these achievements reinforces your commitment to intermittent fasting and provides continual motivation.

Create rituals around these celebrations. Perhaps you could have a special meal at the end of each month to celebrate sticking to your fasting goals, or buy yourself a small gift when you reach a significant health milestone. Sharing these achievements with your support network can also amplify the celebratory feeling and encourage others in their fasting journeys.

By integrating these practices - cultivating an adaptive mindset, setting long-term goals, building emotional resilience, and celebrating milestones - you create a robust framework that supports your intermittent fasting lifestyle not just now but for years to come. These strategies ensure that intermittent fasting remains a fulfilling and beneficial part of your life, adapting to your needs and goals as you journey through different stages of life.

When to Reassess Your Fasting Plan

As you continue to integrate intermittent fasting into your lifestyle, it's crucial to stay attuned to the signals your body sends, indicating whether your current fasting regimen remains effective or needs adjustment. Recognizing the signs that warrant a reassessment of your fasting plan is key to maintaining its benefits and ensuring it supports your health at every stage. One clear signal is a change in your health status. If you find yourself feeling unusually fatigued, experiencing digestive discomfort, or noticing changes in your sleep patterns that coincide with your fasting routine, these could be signs that your body is not responding well to your current fasting schedule. Similarly, if you've stopped seeing progress - whether your goal is weight management, improved energy levels, or better blood sugar control - this plateau can be a signal that your body has adapted to the fasting regimen and it might be time for a change. Just eating earlier in the day and fasting earlier, leaving more hours before bed can make a difference.

Another scenario that might prompt a reassessment is a significant lifestyle change. Major life events such as retirement, changes in your work schedule, or shifts in family dynamics can disrupt your routine and may necessitate adjustments to your fasting schedule.

For example, if retirement leads to a more sedentary lifestyle, you might find that a shorter fasting window or more frequent, smaller meals could help manage energy levels and metabolic health more effectively. Conversely, an increase in physical activity might require adjustments to your eating windows to ensure adequate nutrition and recovery. If you are not overweight then some feasting days may reset your metabolism and improve your metabolism and increase energy.

Consulting with healthcare professionals is an essential step in reassessing your fasting plan. A dietitian or a healthcare provider specialising in nutritional medicine can offer valuable insights into how best to adjust your fasting regimen in response to changes in your health status or lifestyle. We can help you understand the underlying causes of any new symptoms and provide guidance on how to modify your fasting plan to better suit your current needs, ensuring that it continues to be safe and effective. This professional guidance is particularly important if you have any chronic health conditions that could be affected by dietary changes.

Feedback Loops

Establishing regular feedback loops is an effective strategy to monitor the success of your fasting plan and make informed adjustments. This could involve maintaining a journal where you record not only your fasting hours and what you eat but also how you feel during different stages of the fasting cycle. Over time, this record can provide insights into patterns that might indicate the need for adjustments. For example, you may notice that you consistently feel lethargic at certain times during your fasting period, suggesting that a change in the timing or composition of your last meal before the fast might be needed.

Technology can also serve as a tool for maintaining feedback loops. Many apps not only track fasting and eating windows but also allow you to log physical symptoms, mood changes, and energy levels. These digital tools can help you correlate specific aspects of your fasting regimen with changes in your well-being, providing a data-driven basis for making adjustments. Moreover, some apps offer community features where you can share experiences and tips with others who are also practising intermittent fasting, providing a broader perspective on potential adjustments and enhancements to your regimen.

Incorporating these strategies - being attentive to signs of needed change, consulting with professionals, and establishing effective feedback mechanisms - ensures that your intermittent fasting regimen remains a dynamic and responsive aspect of your overall health strategy. By regularly assessing and adjusting your approach, you empower yourself to maintain an effective and enjoyable fasting experience that applies to your evolving lifestyle and health needs, ensuring continued benefits and alignment with your personal health goals.

Combining Intermittent Fasting with Other Dietary Theories

In the quest for optimal health, intertwining intermittent fasting with other dietary approaches can magnify the benefits and cater to your specific health needs more holistically. Imagine this integration as creating a symphony with each dietary approach contributing a unique tone, harmonising to enhance your overall health. For instance, combining intermittent fasting with the Mediterranean diet, renowned for its heart-healthy benefits, can provide a robust framework for improving cardiovascular health and overall longevity. The Mediterranean diet, rich in fruits, vegetables, whole grains, and healthy fats, complements intermittent fasting by providing dense nutrients during eating windows, thus maximising the nourishment your body receives during those periods.

Similarly, a plant-based diet, which emphasises foods derived from plants and is typically low in fat and high in fibre, pairs well with intermittent fasting, especially for those looking to improve their weight management and reduce the risk of chronic diseases such as type 2 diabetes. This combination can help regulate blood sugar levels more effectively, as the high fibre content of a plant-based diet slows down glucose absorption, preventing spikes and crashes in blood sugar levels, while the fasting periods help improve insulin sensitivity.

Tailoring these combinations to address specific health concerns can significantly enhance their effectiveness. For example, if heart health is a concern, integrating the Mediterranean diet into your fasting regimen ensures that you consume ample amounts of omega-3 fatty acids, antioxidants, and polyphenols, which are known for their roles in reducing inflammation and oxidative stress, factors associated with heart disease. On the other hand, if cognitive function is your focus, you might find that a plant-based diet rich in fruits, vegetables, and nuts, combined with regular fasting periods, helps to maintain brain health. These foods are loaded with vitamins and antioxidants that protect brain cells from damage while fasting contributes by boosting brain-derived neurotrophic factor (BDNF), a protein that supports the survival of existing neurons and encourages the growth of new neurons and synapses. However the longevity professionals, biologists and professors have postulated that as we age we may need more red meat so listen to your body as well as the scientists.

Balancing nutrient intake is crucial when merging intermittent fasting with other dietary preferences or restrictions. It's important to ensure that you are not only meeting your caloric needs but also getting a well-rounded intake of nutrients. For instance, if you are practising intermittent fasting alongside a vegetarian diet, it's vital to incorporate a variety of protein sources like legumes, nuts, and seeds to compensate for the absence of meat. Additionally, focusing on iron-rich plant foods such as spinach and beans, and pairing them with vitamin C-rich foods like tomatoes and citrus fruits can enhance iron absorption, crucial for preventing anaemia.

Case Studies

To bring these concepts to life, consider the example of Lisa, a 58-year-old who managed to significantly improve her heart health by combining intermittent fasting with the Mediterranean diet. After struggling with high cholesterol and hypertension, Lisa adopted a 16/8 fasting schedule and during her eating windows, she focused on Mediterranean staples like fish, olive oil, and plenty of fresh produce. Over six months, not only did her cholesterol levels and blood pressure drop, but she also experienced a noticeable increase in energy and mental clarity.

Another inspiring case is that of Michael, a 65-year-old diabetic who integrated a plant-based diet with intermittent fasting. By consuming whole, plant-based foods within a 10-hour eating window and fasting for 14 hours, Michael saw a dramatic improvement in his blood sugar control and a reduction in his dependency on insulin. His diet was rich in legumes, whole grains, and vegetables, which helped to stabilise his blood sugar levels throughout the day.

These examples underscore the potential of combining intermittent fasting with tailored dietary approaches to address specific health issues effectively. By thoughtfully selecting and integrating different dietary theories with intermittent fasting, you can create a personalised eating plan that not only aligns with your health goals and dietary preferences but also enhances your quality of life. Whether you're looking to boost heart health, manage diabetes, or simply maintain a healthy weight, the synergy between intermittent fasting and other dietary practices offers a powerful tool for achieving and sustaining optimal health.

The Future of Intermittent Fasting for Seniors

As we look towards the horizon of ageing gracefully, the intersection of intermittent fasting and senior health continues to spark both interest and innovation. Emerging research is increasingly focusing on the nuances of how older adults can adapt and thrive on intermittent fasting regimes, particularly with an eye towards enhancing cognitive health and mobility. Studies are beginning to show that the principles of intermittent fasting, such as enhanced autophagy and improved metabolic efficiency, might significantly benefit cognitive functions. This is particularly promising for seniors, as cognitive decline is a major concern.

The process of autophagy, stimulated by fasting, plays a crucial role in clearing out the protein build-ups associated with degenerative diseases like Alzheimer's and Parkinson's. Moreover, intermittent fasting has been shown to improve the brain's resistance to stress and injury, which could potentially slow down the progression of cognitive decline and enhance the quality of life in one's later years.

Mobility, another critical aspect of senior health, also benefits from the anti-inflammatory and weight management effects of intermittent fasting. Maintaining a healthy weight can significantly reduce the wear and tear on joints and bones, which is crucial for preserving mobility and independence. Furthermore, the boost in human growth hormone (HGH) production, a well-documented effect of intermittent fasting, may help in maintaining muscle strength and mass, which are vital for mobility and overall health. The potential for intermittent fasting to mitigate some of the common age-related declines in muscle and joint function offers a compelling avenue for further research and application in geriatric care.

The integration of technology in managing health regimes like intermittent fasting is a boon, especially for seniors. Wearable devices and mobile apps are becoming indispensable tools in personal health management.

These technologies offer the ability to monitor key health metrics such as blood glucose levels, heart rate, and physical activity, which can help seniors tailor their fasting and activity periods more effectively. Apps designed to track fasting windows and nutritional intake are becoming more user-friendly, making it easier for seniors to maintain their fasting schedules and ensure they are meeting their nutritional needs during eating windows. This tech-savvy approach not only empowers seniors to take charge of their health but also provides caregivers and healthcare providers with real-time data to better support the individual's health goals.

Looking forward, the potential for policy and healthcare integration to support the adoption of intermittent life-long practices among seniors is immense. As healthcare systems increasingly recognize the preventive and therapeutic benefits of lifestyle modifications like intermittent fasting, we may see more initiatives aimed at incorporating these strategies into standard preventive care for seniors. This could include educational programs to inform seniors about the benefits of intermittent fasting, training for healthcare providers on how to guide older adults through the process safely, and even the integration of fasting protocols in community senior health programs.

Such developments would not only broaden the accessibility of intermittent fasting for seniors but also support its implementation as a part of holistic health maintenance and disease prevention.

In preparing for future health challenges, maintaining flexibility and adaptability in one's fasting practices remains crucial. As the body ages, its responses to fasting can change, necessitating adjustments to the regimen to continue reaping the benefits without compromising overall health. Regular health assessments to monitor how the body is responding to fasting, along with adjustments to diet and fasting schedules, can help mitigate risks and enhance the efficacy of the practice. For seniors, this might mean shorter fasting periods or modified eating windows that align better with their energy needs and metabolic capabilities.

Ensuring a personalised approach that respects the unique health profiles and lifestyles of older adults will be key in safely and effectively extending the benefits of intermittent fasting across the lifespan. In Russia there was a clinic that had many over 80s doing long fasts albeit with supervision so I am of the opinion that it is perfectly safe for seniors to fast. They are wise enough to be aware of what their body is telling them.

As we continue to explore and understand the full spectrum of intermittent fasting's benefits, its role in supporting senior health through enhanced cognitive function, improved mobility, and integrated technology use is promising.

The future of intermittent fasting for seniors looks not only hopeful but also revolutionary, offering new pathways to ageing with health, dignity, and vitality.

Leaving a Legacy of Health: Teaching IF to the Next Generation

When we think about the legacy we wish to leave behind, our minds often turn to tangible assets. However, one of the most impactful legacies we can provide is that of health - specifically, educating our families about the benefits and practices of intermittent fasting. Introducing this lifestyle to different age groups within your family not only promotes healthier generations but also fosters an environment where health and wellness are prioritised. When teaching intermittent fasting to the family, it's crucial to tailor the discussion to age-appropriate levels. For younger members, this might mean simple explanations about why eating times are structured and the benefits it brings, such as better concentration or energy. Older family members might be more receptive to discussions about the specific health benefits, such as weight management or improved metabolic health.

Children and teenagers, in particular, are at a formative stage where lifelong habits begin to set. Children need to eat healthy meals but should be discouraged from snacking. By incorporating the principles of intermittent fasting in ways that don't feel restrictive - such as focusing on delaying breakfast to accommodate a more natural eating window - you subtly instil habits that can lead to long-term health benefits. It's about framing intermittent fasting as a positive, empowering choice rather than a restriction, which can help inculcate these habits without resistance. For adult family members, especially those who might be sceptical or set in their dietary ways, sharing your personal experiences, backed by scientific research, can be more persuasive. Discussing how intermittent fasting has improved your energy levels, weight management, and overall vitality might encourage them to try it themselves.

Leading by example is one of the most powerful methods of teaching. When family and friends see the positive changes in your health and lifestyle as a result of intermittent fasting, it naturally piques their interest. This approach is less about preaching the benefits and more about embodying them.

When you navigate your health journey with visible positivity and results, it sends a compelling message to your loved ones about the effectiveness of intermittent fasting. This method of influence is subtle yet powerful, as the changes they observe in you can motivate them to adopt similar habits.

Creating resources and guides can further extend your influence and help in educating others about intermittent fasting. Whether it's a simple handout that outlines the basics, a blog sharing your personal journey and tips, or a more comprehensive guidebook that delves into the scientific underpinnings and methods of intermittent fasting, these resources can be invaluable. They serve as accessible references that people can turn to for information and guidance. Additionally, consider creating or distributing meal planners, recipes, or even a FAQ document to help beginners ease into the practice of intermittent fasting with more confidence and support. Also consider leaving an insightful review of this book to help people understand that IF is very helpful to them. The author would like to advise that pregnant and lactating women of your acquaintance should be encouraged to eat healthy but probably not fast.

Community engagement is another powerful avenue for spreading knowledge and enthusiasm about intermittent fasting. Participating in or organising workshops, talks, or informal meet-ups can not only educate but also build a community of like-minded individuals who support each other. These gatherings can be particularly effective in demystifying intermittent fasting for those who might be intimidated by the idea or unsure of how to start. Moreover, your active involvement in promoting health and wellness can inspire others in your community to take their health into their own hands, potentially leading to a wider adoption and normalisation of intermittent fasting.

By taking these steps - educating your family, leading by example, creating helpful resources, and engaging with the community - you do more than just share a lifestyle. You instil values of health and wellness that can ripple through generations, creating a legacy that extends far beyond your own life. This approach not only enhances the lives of your loved ones but also contributes to a broader cultural shift towards health consciousness. As you continue to advocate for intermittent fasting and its benefits, you help pave the way for healthier communities, influenced by the knowledge and practices you've shared.

In summary, this chapter has explored how your intermittent fasting journey can influence and benefit not just you but your family and wider community. By educating younger generations, setting a positive example, creating useful resources, and engaging in community activities, you foster a broader understanding and adoption of intermittent fasting. This collective approach not only multiplies the benefits of intermittent fasting but also helps ensure its sustainability and relevance for future generations. As we move forward, let us consider how we can continue to adapt and advocate for practices that support our collective health and well-being.

Conclusion

As we draw this guide to a close, let us reflect on the transformative journey we've embarked on together through the pages of this book. From debunking long-held myths that often discourage fasting among older women, to providing a comprehensive and adaptable roadmap for integrating intermittent fasting into your life, we've covered significant ground. The benefits of intermittent fasting, such as enhanced metabolic health, effective weight management, improved hormonal balance, and increased longevity, are not just theoretical but practical and attainable.

With my expertise as a naturopath specialising in allergies, fasting, and weight loss, combined with my personal journey through the challenges of maintaining health and managing weight post-menopause, I've strived to offer you not just information, but a perspective rooted in both professional knowledge and personal experience. This dual vantage point aims to reassure and guide you as you navigate your own path towards better health.

Remember, starting an intermittent fasting lifestyle involves selecting a fasting plan that resonates with your daily routine, integrating essential nutritional needs, and being willing to adapt these as you age.

It's crucial to listen to your body and consult healthcare professionals to tailor this approach to your individual health requirements, especially if you are managing health conditions or taking medications.

Intermittent fasting is not a quick fix but a profound journey of discovery and adaptation. It requires patience and resilience, with benefits that accumulate and become more apparent over time. Embrace this path not just for weight management but for a revitalised sense of well-being and empowerment over your own health.

I encourage you to take that first step towards integrating intermittent fasting into your lifestyle. Connect with support groups, engage in online communities, or attend local meetups with other women who are on the same journey. Sharing your experiences and challenges, and celebrating your successes with others can be incredibly rewarding and motivating.

In closing, I share with you a personal note of encouragement and solidarity. My hope is that this book serves as a catalyst for your own transformative journey, just as intermittent fasting has been for me. Together, let us embrace the potential for a healthier, more vibrant life as we continue to grow and thrive.

This book was written with a goal in mind: to empower you, women over 50, to take control of your health and well-being through the practice of intermittent fasting. Backed by science, enriched by personal experience, and attuned to the unique challenges and opportunities that come with age, I hope it inspires you to see your later years as a time of healthful rejuvenation.

Thank you for joining me on this journey. Let's continue to support each other and move forward with strength and confidence. Here's to our health, longevity, and happiness!

References

- *How intermittent fasting affects female hormones*
  https://www.sciencedaily.com/releases
- *Hallmarks of Aging: An Autophagic Perspective*
- *Best Intermittent Fasting App Of 2024,*
  https://www.womenshealthmag.com/weight-loss/g29554400/intermittent-fasting-apps/
- *The Definitive Guide to Healthy Eating in Your 50s and 60s*
  https://www.healthline.com/nutrition/healthy-eating-50s-
- *Intermittent fasting: Researchers debunk 4 common myths*
  https://www.medicalnewstoday.com/articles/intermittent-fasting-myths-debunked
- *Intermittent Fasting for Menopause: What You Need to ...*
  https://drbrighten.com/intermittent-fasting-for-menopause/
- *Phytoestrogens: Benefits, risks, and food list*
  https://www.medicalnewstoday.com/articles/320630
- *Managing menopause symptoms with nutrition and diet*
  https://www.nutrition.org.uk/nutrition-for/women/menopause/managing-menopause-symptoms-with-nutrition-and-diet/
- *Effect of Intermittent Fasting on Reproductive Hormones*
  https://www.ncbi.nlm.nih.gov/
- *Intermittent Fasting for Menopause: What You Need to Know*
  https://drbrighten.com/intermittent-fasting-for-menopause/
- *Slow down - and try mindful eating - Harvard Health*
  https://www.health.harvard.edu/staying-healthy/slow-downand-try-mindful-eating
- *Is intermittent fasting safe for older adults?*
  https://www.health.harvard.edu/staying-healthy/is-intermittent-fasting-safe-for-older-adults
- *Getting past a weight-loss plateau - Mayo Clinic*
  https://www.mayoclinic.org/healthy-lifestyle/weight-loss/in-depth/weight-loss-plateau/art-2004

- *Intermittent Fasting Enhanced the Cognitive Function in Older Adults with Mild Cognitive Impairment by Inducing Biochemical and Metabolic Health*
  https://www.ncbi.nlm.nih.gov/pmc/articles
- *Mindful Eating - The Nutrition Source*
  https://nutritionsource.hsph.harvard.edu/mindful-eating/
- *Exercise beyond menopause: Dos and Don'ts -*
  https://www.ncbi.nlm.nih.gov/pmc/articles/
- *Fast and Fluid: The Benefits of Hydration During Fasting*
  https://www.medanta.org
- *The Effects of Intermittent Fasting on Brain and Cognition*
- *Intermittent fasting in the prevention and treatment of cancer*
  https://acsjournals.onlinelibrary.wiley.com
- *Intermittent fasting is safe, effective for those with Type 2 Diabetes*
  https://today.uic.edu/intermittent-fasting-diabetes-weight-loss/
- *How one woman used intermittent fasting to lose 80 pounds*
  https://www.nbcnews.com/better/lifestyle/how-one-woman-used-intermittent-fasting-lose-80-pounds
- *Can the Keto Diet Help with Menopause? - Healthline*
  https://www.healthline.com/nutrition/keto-and-menopause
- *Effect of Intermittent Fasting on Reproductive Hormones.*
  https://www.ncbi.nlm.nih.gov/pmc/articles
- *What Midlife Women Should Know About Intermittent Fasting*
  https://www.everydayhealth.com/womens-health/what-midlife-women-should-know-about-intermittent-fasting/

Printed in Dunstable, United Kingdom